DRAGON
FIRE
PRODUCTIONS

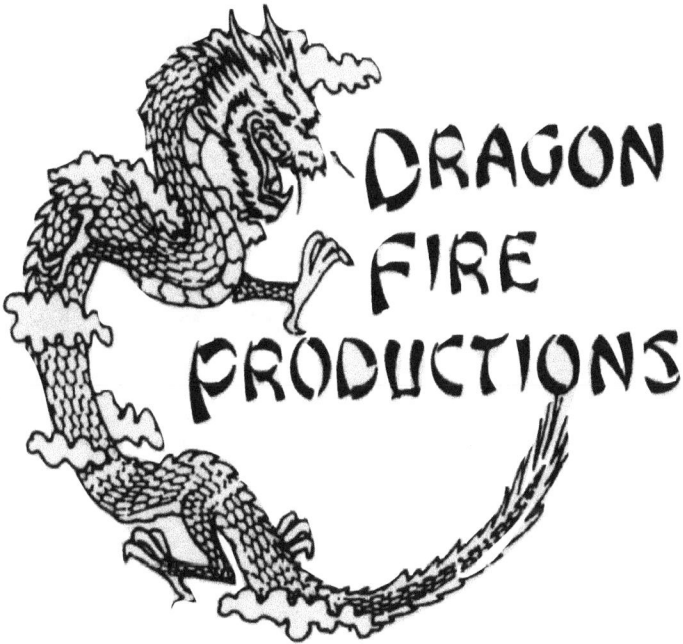

The Mountain Path, by Caryn Boyd Diel

Bellingham, Washington

© 2019

THE
MOUNTAIN PATH

Taoist Healing with Chi Nei Tsang

Caryn Boyd Diel

Printed in the United States of America

First Printing, 2019

Cover Design & Photography by © Caryn Boyd Diel
Cover images taken at the Huashan mountain in China.

Book design by © Rachel Johnson

The Mountain Path/ Caryn Diel. -- 1st ed.
ISBN 9781733869508

Acknowledgements

I would like to thank Mui Wattanaba for sharing his gift of healing with Master Mantak Chia. And I also thank Gilles Marin, my first CNT instructor, who inherited this knowledge from Master Mantak Chia. Many students and clients of mine have received benefit from this information, and have allowed me to share my enthusiasm for this an ancient art form. I have been changed as a result of learning and receiving CNT treatments over the years. And I have reconnected with ancient Taoist healing as a result of my further studies into the realm of traditional Chinese medicine. One of my I Ching teachers, Juan Li, would say that this is a fulfillment of my destiny, and that is, indeed, how it feels to me.

Foreword

The digestive system is ancient, the most ancient system in our body, and as such the organs are a current record of our evolutionary status on this planet. In the last 500 years of life on earth a lot has changed in our environment, our working and living situations, and the foods that we eat. There are more toxins, and a faster pace of life. Our bodies are struggling to adapt to this changing environment, as is witnessed from the many new diseases and digestive problems that plague humanity. Our digestion is especially challenged with the food choices we have available and the ways in which these foods are grown.

Chi Nei Tsang treatments have both direct and indirect results. The physical human touch can relieve tension and improve digestion. The secondary indirect result may be a resolution of emotions that were stored in the body.

Chi Nei Tsang sessions can bring the body into the present moment in a clear and refreshed state that allows for more authentic interactions. The body often becomes unhampered so that life can unfold with more ease.

This is an ancient healing modality, and no doubt, there were distractions and tensions that ancient peoples dealt with. We only have to read the ancient texts to see that people 1000, 2000 and 4000 years ago had situations that required their attention and often resulted in emotional imbalances. It is indeed a joyful expe-rience to connect with humans from long ago through this healing modality and to know that we have in our hands a healing practice that is still applicable today.

This book is dedicated to our Ancestors.

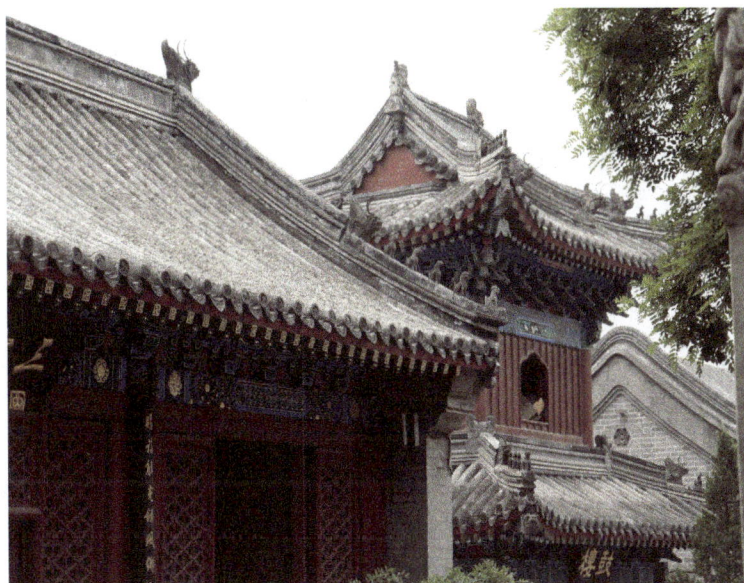

Contents

The Mountain Path

Caryn Boyd Diel

The Mountain Path

As we walk the mountain path we become aware of the interdependence of all things. Trees, sky, rock, fungi, sun, rivers, clouds, lakes, plants, animals, rain, humanity. Nature finds its own balance within space and time. Taoists in Japan and China worship the mountains, the birthplace of rivers. Temples and places of peaceful contemplation are plentiful in the mountains. Shugendo is the name for mountain worship in Japan. A path of self-enlightenment, similar to that of hermits and mountain sages in China, the practice of Shugendo included seclusion, meditation and fasting. In China, there are five sacred mountains; Songshan in the center, Taishan in the East, Hengshan in the north, Huashan in the west and Nanyue in the south. Pilgrimage is done in a specific order to open the energies of the mountains.

For many of us, the mountain path begins wide and many others are standing and walking along side of us. Yet, if you have ever walked a high mountain path you know that the path often becomes narrow and winding and only one foot will fit in front of the other. Concentration is required to stay sure footed and focused in order to reach the top. Only a few others are encountered on mountain paths, and those who join us often walk in silence. The sound of earth and stone and dry leaves underfoot mark the pace at which we ascend. Each breath becomes measured. Many seek the heightened perspectives gained at the top of the mountain.

The Trigram for Mountain is the symbol of meditation and structure. One yang line on the top and two yin lines beneath.

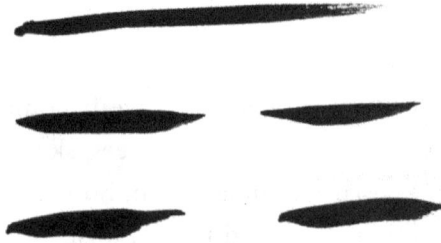

Trigram for Mountain

In times past, travelers passed through hand crafted mountain gates of decorated wood and stone, which opened the path ahead. The gates were a symbolic opening of the way, a conscious stepping over into the next phase of the journey, a necessary tribute to the wisdom held by the mountain. Sometimes a gatekeeper would record the comings and goings of the pilgrim. Many of life's passages are like this, there is a record of our destiny and the necessary initiations of the journey we call life.

The Mountain Path represents the highest of spiritual goals in most traditions. Making a pilgrimage to the mountain has become a symbol of inner commitment to a higher purpose, and to goals that transcend beyond life. At each crossing there is a new vista, but the ultimate goal is to reach above it all and rest at the top, with no need to take one more step – the accomplishment of a lifetime, or many lifetimes of effort, has come to an end. At that moment in our journey when our gaze is firmly focused on the goal, we must become even more diligent and cautious, watching every step, careful not to slip off of the mountain.

The Mountain Path is not for everyone as it requires deep inner commitment and the ability to be in silence with oneself, surrendering to the dizzying heights and rarified air of the mountain peaks. Leaving behind any comforts, the one embarking on the mountain path must realize that after seeing from higher perspectives, one does not come back the same as before. The mountain changes those who wait to hear her secrets. The mountain tops open us to higher vision and knowing, and bring us closer to the heavens. The movement of stars becomes fixed within our mind's eye, and it is from our inner galaxy that we see out into the world of human experiences.

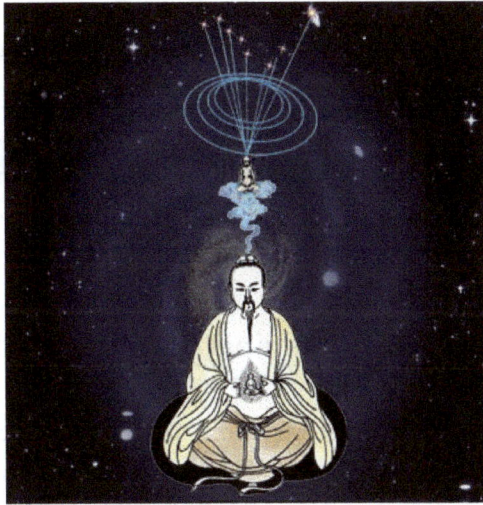

As an ancient shamanic practice, Taoism leads one onto the mountain path of embodied spirituality. For thousands of years, practitioners have sought the stillness and quiet of mountain sanc-tuaries in which to perfect their alchemical practices. No need to leave the body to have a spiritual experience, as the refined al-chemical practices merged the etheric dimensions with physical matter to allow for the heightened experience of humanity.

A Migration Story

The story of Abdominal Massage is a story of temple practice and migration, perhaps reaching back into India 10,000 years ago. Chinese Anmo massage migrated to Japan to become Anma, with the specialty of Ampuku – abdominal massage taking hold and thriving in Japan during the 6th century. Physician and Warrior Monks carried the information from China through Korea and into Japan.

The story of Chi Nei Tsang, Anmo, Anma, Ampuku and of many other healing traditions is a story of the migrations of its people. People around the planet have migrated to find food and shelter, to discover new places, and to seek safety in times of political turmoil. Some migrated for the pure joy of exploration, others to seek a safe haven.

History of Abdominal Massage in China

"Anmo has played an important role in the practice of medicine in China since ancient times. Archeologists, studying the inscriptions found on bones and tortoise shells used in divination practice, have found references to massage treatment for illnesses written in jiaguwen, the earliest extant form of writing in China, dating back to as early as the Shang Dynasty (16th-11th centuries BC). For example, on one such bone a question is inscribed: "Can the querent's abdominal pain be successfully treated with massage?" Another asks whether or not a certain female massage practitioner named Zao can cure an illness and thus should be sent for." Matthew Miller l.ac article and records from the Shanghai Science and Technology Press, 1983-1984.

Mawangdui is an archaeological site which was uncovered in 1963 near Changsha in the Hunan province of southeastern China. It is the burial place of a high-ranking official, the marquess of Dai, who lived in the 2nd century BC, and of his immediate family. He was a noble who governed small semiautonomous domains during the Han dynasty. The tombs were discovered during the construction of a hospital. During the excavation of the Ma Wang Dui tomb (dated 168 BC) numerous medical texts on silk scrolls and bamboo strips were unearthed. Many of these (including Fifty-two Medical Formulas, Illustrated Health Exercises, Health Preservation Formulas, Formulas for Miscellaneous Illnesses and Concerning the Way of Everything Under Heaven) contain references to Anmo, gymnastics and breathing exercises. The Fifty-two Medical Formulas contains references to specific Anmo techniques such as compression (an), gliding (mo), scratching (sao), scraping (gua), rubbing (fu) and percussing (ji).

From the Three Kingdoms period (ad 220-280) up until the Tang Dynasty (ad 618-907), the imperial medical schools included Anmo as a specialized branch of medicine. Practitioners who specialized in Anmo during the Tang dynasty were divided into three levels: Anmo doctorates, Anmo masters and Anmo technicians. At that time, the scope of the Anmo specialty included therapeutic gymnastics and orthopedics (bone-setting).

The Huangdi Qipo Anmo is supposedly the earliest Chinese medical text devoted entirely to the practice of Anmo. The Huangdi Nei Jing, the Yellow Emperor's Inner Classic is the earliest surviving canonical text of traditional Chinese medicine. Anmo is referred to in 30 different chapters of the Nei Jing. In one chapter, Anmo is said to have originated in the central area of China (Henan, Luoyang). Elsewhere, Anmo is indicated for the treatment of various disorders, including joint pain, muscle weakness, facial paralysis and stomach pain.

It was also at this time that Chinese Anmo was first brought to Korea, Japan and other Asian countries where separate developments began such as Japanese amma and shiatsu.

Sun Simiao, the famous Chinese physician, recommended that after meals one should massage the abdomen with warm hands and go out for a stroll. He wrote that this would help digestion and "prevent a hundred illnesses."

Anmo suffered its share of setbacks during the tumultuous years of the twentieth century. Perhaps the greatest blow was dealt during the Nationalist period (1911-1949) when the government led a campaign against traditional Chinese medicine. In 1936, the government announced that "traditional medicine has no scientific foundation" and its practice was banned. During this time, very few physicians went into Anmo practice. Nevertheless, Anmo continued to be a popular form of healing among the common people, and its techniques were preserved outside the halls of officially-sanctioned medical practice.

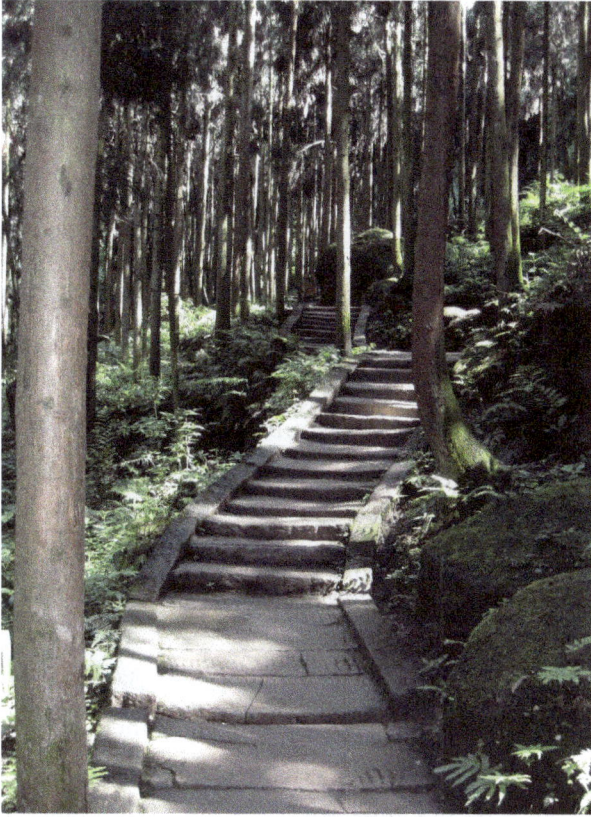

A mountain path in China.

Migration to Japan

Migrations of physician monks from China to Japan during the 5th, 6th, and 7th centuries introduced Taoist immortality practices and Chinese Medicine practices such as Anmo. Migrations from China to Thailand and Vietnam brought concepts of traditional Chinese medicine like acupuncture, moxibustion, herbal medicine and AnMo massage. Later migrations from India, Burma, and Southern China brought new concepts of healing into Thailand. The Sen Sib meridians used in Thai massage arrived from India and found their way into the medical records of the Wat Pho in Bangkok. TokSen from Burma found its way to Tao Gardens in Thailand.

The massage practices of Anmo/Anma are the foundation of Oriental medicine. Su Wen and Ling Shu were written to describe many concepts of Oriental medicine. Here we see references to Anmo massage. In about 2600 BC in China, The Yellow Emperor Huang Di collaborated on the Yellow Emperor's Classic of Internal Medicine. Through a series of conversations with his ministers about heaven, man, the earth and their relationships, the Yellow Emperor's classic was written. Schools of medicine were established and hundreds of written texts followed.

Many civil wars in China after this time encouraged the migration of people and information toward Japan. In 1929, acupuncture and traditional medicine were outlawed in China with the rise of Western medicine.

Today, Anma is an integral part of Japanese culture and health care, like a Japanese art form. Anma can be translated as pressing and rubbing, or to spread peace by rubbing. In the past, one had to train for three years in Anma (to become an Anmashi, or massage therapist) before beginning any other medical training. Since most oriental medicine is based on prevention and balancing and restoring health to the internal organs, hand techniques such as Anmo and Anma were taught first to bring hand sensitivity to medical practitioners. Palpation was taught as a high art form with the purpose of diagnosing symptoms and diseases. Historically most people were farmers and craftsmen. Monks had time to refine their healing and meditation practices in the solitude of the mountain monasteries, far from the cities.

Anma massage training includes spiritual practice and meditation. Methods of Anpuku (abdominal massage) were developed by Shinsai Ota in the 17th century.

Many techniques are documented in the writings of Mochizuki and Kiiko Matsumoto. Anpuku translates as to ease the hara, or abdomen. Anpuku is a separate discipline from AnMa massage, and it requires special training. The history of Anpuku therapy can be traced back to the Nara and Heian periods in Japan (AD 710-1185).

"Anma is part of Oriental Medicine and the development of Anpuku was very closely related to Fukushin (which is abdominal diagnosis in Oriental medicine and acupuncture). Fukushin originated in China, along with acupuncture methods, and, after it emigrated to Japan, developed and became a very important diagnostic method in Japanase acupuncture. As with Anpuku, Fukushin also became more well developed and widely practiced during the Edo period. In China, though, Fukushin did not develop as it did in Japan, and in modern times, seems to have died out and been succeeded by tongue diagnosis." (Mochizuki, 340)

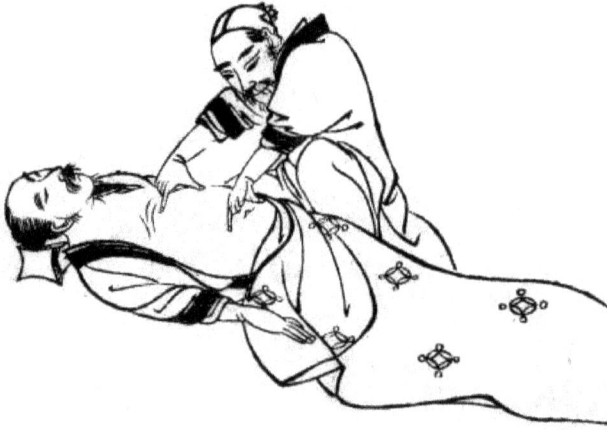

Kenbiki Ho - Point Rocking Method

Anpuku Zukai

(Illustrated Manual of Abdominal Massage) written by Shinsai Ota in 1827.

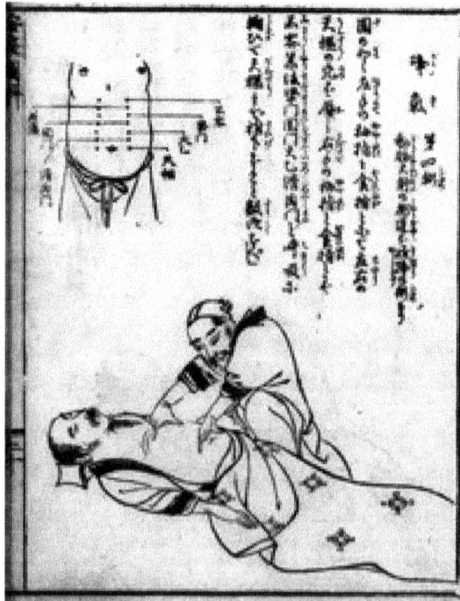

Anpuku technique: Konki (descending energy) method of adjusting the Ki of the abdomen.

"Anma is one of the oldest forms of massage methods in the world and the first form of massage recorded in textbook form that still exists today. It is unknown just how long ago Anma began to be practiced but it is likely at least 5,000 years and it might even go back as far as 10,000 years. Anma became a written system of massage and treatment over 2,500 years ago." (Mochizuki, 7)

"During the fifth century, monks travelled from China to Japan bringing their religion and medical knowledge with them." (Mochizuki, 8)

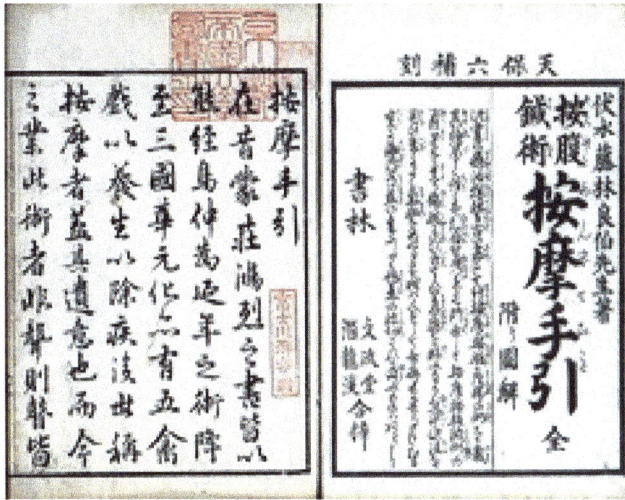

Introduction page of the Anma Tebiki

Anmo Receives a New Name

Mantak Chia was born in Thailand in 1944 to Chinese parents who had left China. In his 30's, in 1976, Master Chia, with his wife and son, moved to New York, a safe haven for many people post Viet Nam War, and safe from Japanese invasions of Thailand. Master Mantak Chia says he met Dr. Mui when he was twenty. His uncle needed healing for his shoulder, and at that time, Dr. Mui was performing healings in Thailand. After successfully treating his uncle, Master Chia studied with Dr. Mui for several years, learning what he could by observing. Mantak Chia was an eager student; a young man who would study and bring a healing art to the Western world.

He re-named an ancient healing practice that he had learned from his teacher, Mui Wattanaba, calling it Chi Nei Tsang – internal organ massage, or moving chi into the organs. We may surmise from his name that Mui Wattanaba is from Japanese ancestry, although the story is that Dr Mui came from a long line of healers who left China. Mantak Chia introduced Chi Nei Tsang to a small group in New York City during the 1970's and 1980's. To this day, many of his students are still teaching and practicing Chi Nei Tsang (CNT) and the other Healing Tao meditations that he taught.

My Personal Migration

I moved to Santa Fe from Hawaii in 1995 to study Energy Medicine with Barbara Brennan. At the time, her school of Energy Medicine was in NYC, and it was easier for me to travel to NYC from Santa Fe than Hawaii. In 1998 I received a Thai massage in Santa Fe. The masseuses finished with a powerful touch to my navel. I sensed a strong energy and asked her what it she had done. She said this was part of her training in Chi Nei Tsang and led me to her teacher, Gilles Marin. Gilles, whose parents are French and Vietnamese, had moved from France in 1980 to San Francisco, and in 1983 went to study with Mantak Chia in the Catskill mountains of upstate New York. I went immediately to study with Gilles. He was teaching a CNT class in Santa Cruz at the Land of the Medicine Buddha. My life changed course, guided by my belly.

This is where my story begins. Already in my fortics, I had enough training in several fields to last a lifetime, but Chi Nei Tsang seemed to be the missing link, and indeed opened my memory to lifetimes in China and Taoist healing. I studied with Gilles Marin, and later with Mantak Chia who had returned to live at Tao Gardens in Thailand. Fortunately for me, Juan Li, a close friend and illustrator for Mantak Chia, was also living in Santa Fe at this time. I studied Taoist meditation and the I Ching with Juan Li. Juan, born in Cuba to a father from China and a mother from Cuba, had fled from to New York City, where he met Mantak Chia. The only things that Juan was able to take with him from

Cuba were three Chinese coins from his father which he hid in the spine of a book the Communist Manifesto.

When Gilles encouraged me to start teaching, I had no idea what the future would bring. I was very enthusiastic and in the year 2000 insisted that all of my clients experience Chi Nei Tsang. I began teaching Chi Nei Tsang in Santa Fe and in 2001 I wanted a name for my budding school. After spending a day looking at the brilliant white clouds in the blue Santa Fe skies, I decided on the White Cloud Institute. Years later I discovered that there was a White Cloud Monastery in Bejing, and a Taoist teacher, One Cloud (Yi Eng), who had taught Taoist meditation to Mantak Chia. One Cloud was gifted by the teachings of a cave dwelling hermit on Mt. Changbai in China – White Cloud. Certainly I was being inspired, but why and by whom? My destiny began to unfold rapidly.

I have been on a very focused path for the past 22 years since I arrived in Santa Fe. My spiritual growth became deep and wide like a giant redwood. The White Cloud Institute and its teachings have taken me around the world. Many gifted teachers have come to White Cloud Institute and shared their wisdom. The information is still unfolding under my hands. I currently live in Bellingham, Washington where I enjoy walking under the tall cedar trees and teaching Taoist practices. I continue to offer Chi Nei Tsang treatments to clients and the White Cloud Institute continues to offer classes to both the public and seasoned practitioners around the world.

Chi Nei Tsang:
Ancient and Extraordinary Healing

Chi Nei Tsang is simple and profound. The evolution of our organs is tied to the dynamic movement of the elements, plants, minerals, seasons, and the creative energies of the planet.

There are few opportunities in one's life to step into a healing practice and contribute something personal. This is where I feel I am; I have stepped into the river of Taoist healing practices and continue to pull through a stream of information from the past.

What began for me as working around the navel and healing through the belly, has developed into a full grown practice of meditation, qigong, hands on healing, and a point of view which prepares me to deal with life and a transition beyond life.

Chi Nei Tsang is the art and practice of working with the internal organs and the entire being, beginning with deepening the breath and working around the navel. If you can imagine the deepest, most profound sense of rest and safety you can feel in the physical body, then you begin to get a sense of the healing that happens with Chi Nei Tsang.

As a model of healing, Chi Nei Tsang is couched within an ancient history of Taoist practices. My intuition tells me that Anmo/Anma/Chi Nei Tsang were inspired on the mountain tops of Japan and China in monasteries. Chinese Medicine during the past 5,000 to 7,000 years was in held high regards for its ability to diagnose disease and restore health. The Yellow Emperor's conversations with his ministers explored the health of the internal organs, their relationships to nature and the seasons, and the needs of the viscera in great detail and accuracy.

Current day writings depict this type of abdominal massage as a way to free one's body from physical symptoms and emotional distractions in order to be fully present for life. Also, there is growing scientific evidence of the importance of the enteric nervous system – our second brain, the gut. (The Second Brain, Michael Gershon). Kiiko Matsumoto gives excellent descriptions of Hara diagnosis and treatment in his book, Hara Diagnosis, Reflections on the Sea. And Mochizuki gives us five hand techniques for abdominal massage, Ampuku, in his book, Anma, the art of Japanese Massage.

CNT is now emerging as a powerful healing modality. Thanks to the dedication of Mantak Chia and his students, Chi Nei Tsang – Taoist Abdominal Massage – has spread around the world at a time when we desperately need to keep up with the human activities that strain the peace of our body and mind.

Origins of Abdominal Massage

Originating in the shamanic Taoist world thousands of years ago, many indigenous Taoist practices have gone underground or exited China. There is a saying that when things get tough, the Tao hides. Due to the strength of timeless alchemical practices which are available in this lineage, CNT abdominal massage is now gaining respect in the Western world and fits easily into our new understanding of Quantum Energy Healing: awareness = change.

From pure source energies, the Tao arose, a path, a star-based lineage anchored in the Pole Star, moving through the big dipper and onto the planet Earth. Ancient masters observed our place in the universe and refined ways to develop the spiritual body within the physical human form.

Abdominal massage – Chi Nei Tsang – taps into the electromagnetic evolution of organs in the physical body and anchors them deeply into the planet. Qigong and Taoist alchemical meditations also prepare the etheric/spiritual – primordial energy – bodies for transition. I call this embodied enlightenment. It is unusual to find this marriage of heaven and earth in healing practices. CNT also utilizes old healing archetypes of matter, time and space, sound, color, light, pulse, rhythm, the elements, gravity, and sacred geometry. It is ancient and timeless and at the same time an evolutionary model of healing.

For some, a CNT treatment is the first time they have felt at home in the density of earth's atmosphere and in their own physical body. A CNT practitioner, through grounded awareness and practice, can use sound to break up stagnation in the organs, project color to tonify the cells of the body, and tap into the power of the Eight Trigrams and Baqua to give balance to the client.

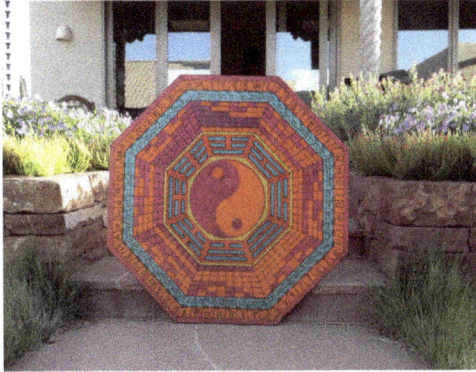

I Ching Bagua designed and created by Keith Waters of Santa Fe.
An example of Sacred Geometry that originated 8000 years ago in China from the vision of FuXi, and later evolved by Shao Yong

What is Chi?

Where does Chi come from? Chi is universal energy, sometimes called the breath that unites all of us. Our bodies transform Chi into life force. Without Chi there is no alchemical process, no life in the body. The Chi emanating from Qigong Masters' hands has been measured and duplicated into Chi machines and sold to the public. A machine cannot produce the same result as two live Chi fields interacting to create change. Chi is as present as the ocean waters are to fish. We are surrounded by it all the time.

Chi may become more charged by pure sunlight, sounds, clean waters, flowers blooming, meditation, Tai Chi and Qigong practices, etc. Chi can be cultivated with these practices for healing others and the self. This is a basic premise of Taoist practices. One may cultivate Chi, store it, circulate it, purify it for self-healing, and emit chi from our hands for healing others.

Many chi cultivating practices are taught in CNT classes to support the work of each practitioner. Foundation practices include the Inner Smile, six healing sounds, bone breathing qigong, fusion of the five elements, and the microcosmic orbit meditation.

There is a quality and quantity of Chi available at all times. Our thoughts and emotions can affect both, and therefore, will affect the health or disease process in our bodies. CNT practitioners need to be disciplined and refresh their chi on a daily basis. The food and water we ingest contribute to our body's vital chi. Our thoughts and emotions must be of a high vibration, our movements must be harmonious and our lives kept in balance. We assume the position of modern-day monks, for whom the practice of hands on healing came to us from physicians and warrior monks of ancient times.

Healing Cycles and the Five Elements

In line with traditional Chinese medicine, we work with the Five Elements: Earth, metal, water, wood, and fire. Using the five elements as a healing model we say that healing begins with an experience of safety provided by earth, and then moves forward with the courage afforded by metal. Healing proceeds as a cycle that we complete when enough momentum exists to propel us forward. Listen to what is said and look at what is happening in your own body and with your clients. Emotions and physical symptoms will guide you to the organ/element that is out of balance.

The five elements are applied in many ways. We can apply their attributes to healing by saying that the Earth element offers us unconditional support. When Earth is strong, we feel supported, nurtured, and have a strong sense of self-esteem. Earth gives one the feeling of safety that is needed to initiate healing. It is from the safety of Earth that we begin and to Earth that we return to accept and integrate healing into our daily lives. A weakness of our Earth element is seen as excessive worry, anxiety, mistrust, insecurity, and poor judgment. The organs that represent Earth are the stomach and pancreas.

Using the Five Elements as a cycle of healing, one begins from the safety of Earth and graduates to the courage of metal. Metal allows us to feel our feelings, gives us the maturity to have discernment, and encourages us to let go of what is no longer needed. As most of us know, we need to feel safe and supported in order to muster the courage to feel what oftentimes seems to be an overwhelming life circumstance. The metal element affords us the courage to cut through situations and let go.

As we become aware of our emotions during a CNT treatment, when there is safety and courage, we can quickly let go of what we no longer need, as if cut by an invisible sword. The honesty and courage to name what is inside is now available to us for healing. Without the courage of metal we shrink away in grief, sadness, and depression, creating symptoms of the lungs and large intestine, such as asthma and constipation; examples of undigested emotions that are held too long in the body.

Beyond our courage and discernment is an ability to trust, regenerate, and create. These virtues represent the water element. Once the emotions are cleared, we move into the mystery of healing and the inspiration of creating new experiences for ourselves. With courage we can move into the mysteries associated with the water element. Water is gentle, yet powerful. It moves effortlessly and humbly. In order to heal deeply we must move into a place of truly recreating ourselves from the sacred depths of water.

Nurturing our kidneys, the most yin organ in the body, with pure water has been a way of healing in all cultures for all times. Higher vibrations of chi will elevate the quality of water in our bodies. When our water element is in balance, we are able to go with the flow and deeply trust the will of the universe. Water gives us the depth of intuition and understanding. Here is where the mystery of healing happens. As we suspend any thinking or judgement, we allow the body to flow forward on its journey. We simply trust. Water gives rise to the growth of the wood element

Wood gives us the upward surge of growth needed to move beyond the present moment. We can use this healthy movement to try new things and think new thoughts. Wood gives us the ability to heal old wounds and grow new branches. Now we are able to bring clarity and momentum to our healing. Wood, which is connected with the liver and gallbladder, brings with it the patience to grow and change. The higher virtues associated with the wood element offer us the ability to treat ourselves with gentleness and kindness throughout the entire process of healing. We have the knowledge now of where to go. Rather than frustration and impatience (the lower vibration of wood), we are clear as to what path to now take

Wood fuels the fire element, our heart, and small intestines. When fire is part of any alchemical change, the change is irreversible, there is no going back. We know in our heart and in our gut that our healing has put us on the right path. With a correct amount of fire, we can digest life, we can digest our food, and we have the passion and inspiration to create and participate fully in life from our hearts. Fire is sometimes the first indication of a change, and there is often no stopping it. Fire creates ashes which fall back to Earth, where we rest again for a while, taking the time to integrate our healing journey. And now we have completed a cycle of change.

The Elements assist us as we walk the Mountain Path.

The five elements represent stages in a cyclical process similar to the changing of the seasons. We are part of nature, and therefore embody the five elements. When our organs are communicating in balance with each other it is a beautiful symphony.

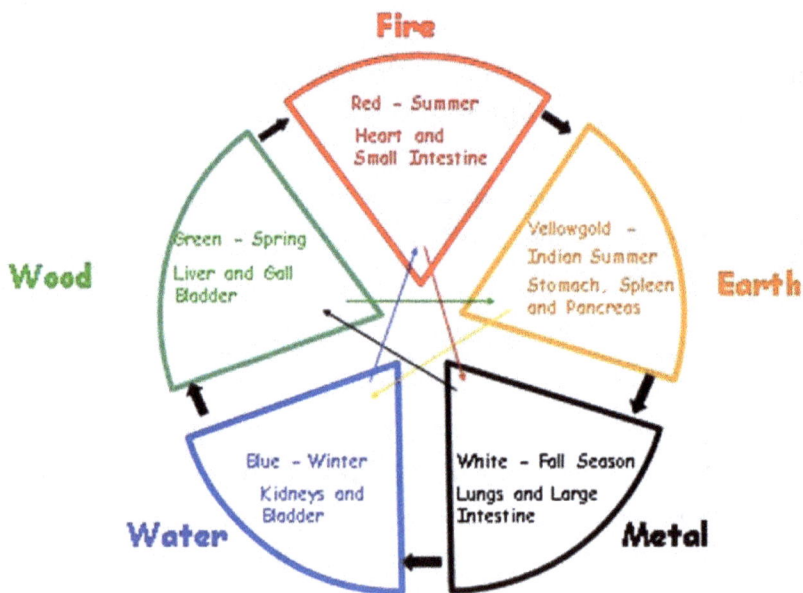

Fire

Red - Summer
Heart and
Small Intestine

Green - Spring
Liver and Gall
Bladder

Wood

Yellowgold -
Indian Summer
Stomach, Spleen
and Pancreas

Earth

Blue - Winter
Kidneys and
Bladder

Water

White - Fall Season
Lungs and Large
Intestine

Metal

Dynamic Movement of the Five Elements

Qigong movements reflect the seasons.

The Metal element, the Season of Autumn moves in a contracting, or gathering in, movement. It is with Metal that we initiate a Chi Nei Tsang treatment. Connecting the breath with the body and letting go of what is no longer needed. Grief and sadness will block forward movement and transformation. When there is contraction there must also be expansion; this is the yin and yang of the Universe. We breathe with Courage.

Water has a sinking action that finds stillness. It is in the depths of Winter that we must find a still place that allows for quiet contemplation and rejuvenation.

Wood moves in an upward and outwardly way, like the sap rising through the branches of trees in early Spring. The liver and gallbladder push toxins and nutrients into the blood.

Fire from the summer sun has the ability to completely expand our chi fields. With the full expansion of fire we can be blessed with the passion and inspiration of our spirit.

Earth brings in the abundance of our harvest; a full cycle of life and healing. The movement of Earth is balanced and brings us into our center. Filling our bellies with a sense of satisfaction and balance.

And so the cycles of the year are reflected in our bodies. And the movements of the seasons are reflected in our Qigong forms. I like to practice Incense Qigong in the fall; it is energetic in its movements and strengthens the breath. In winter I choose a more contemplative form with less movement, finding the stillness of the season and harmonizing my body with the weather.

Treatment Contraindications and Precautions

You may be wondering what, if any, contraindications there are for Chi Nei Tsang treatments. I like to use the word precautions, as there are really no contraindications. The most natural thing to do in response to the distress of another human being is to put your hands on them with the intention of bringing comfort. Therefore, I would encourage you to put your hands on another with a compassionate touch no matter what the condition they are experiencing. You may be able to reduce the pain and stress with a gentle touch so that the physical body begins to heal, as it wants to do.

With respect to basic techniques you are learning and practicing in Chi Nei Tsang, there are some physical conditions that need less vigorous stimulation and more of an energetic touch. Some of these conditions are:

- Bleeding anywhere in the abdomen
- Ulcers
- IUDs
- Hernia
- IBS/SIBO
- Pregnancy
- Pre and Post surgery
- Mesh implants
- Gallstones
- Fibroids
- Cancerous tumors
- Abdominal Aortic Aneurism

- Endometriosis during menstruation
- Post Emergency Room morphine and other pain killers

Touch gently and work indirectly away from the site of con-cern. Healing is a process that requires time in the three dimen-sional world of the body. Each Chi Nei Tsang treatment is unique. What a body needs today will not be the same tomorrow.

Setting the Space For CNT Treatment:

Clear, Ground and Charge

Before you step toward your client to begin a Chi Nei Tsang treatment, take a moment to clear your mind and expand into Primordial Chi. Empty your mind, be in the present moment and expand into the un-manifest creative potential of the void. Feel your feet growing roots into the earth, drawing up Earth energy. Open the crown of your head to the heavens, pulling down heavenly energy. Take a deep breath and relax your belly. Soften your body and mind. Allow the chi to extend out into your hands, keeping your hands soft and sensitive. The Chi that will inform you during the treatment will arise from your client's body and chi field and flow into your hands to be understood. The potential for change and healing resides in your ability to allow chi to flow. The more receptive you are, the more information will come to you. There may not be words to describe the sensations that you feel, however, what is important is that the client is engaged and also feeling their body as it receives CNT.

Begin with the Breath

I like to begin Chi Nei Tsang treatments with a focus on breathing. The breath brings awareness to our self on many levels, and anchors us in the present moment. When we are caught up in our thoughts, we tend to hold our breath, the diaphragm stops moving, and therefore the organs are not moving. If the diaphragm fails, the organs will fail. A healthy abdominal cavity (lower tan tien) has a vibrant amount of internal chi pressure. This keeps the organs and lymph moving without stagnation. Too much pressure is a problem, but more often I see that clients have not enough internal chi pressure to keep the organs healthy. If the lower tan tien is weak and giving little support to the organs, the pelvic floor weakens from excess downward force.

Breathing guides awareness, relaxes the vagus nerve, and builds internal chi pressure with movement of the diaphragm and pelvic floor muscles. Breathing in the lungs (middle tan tien) transforms Chi into Jing (lower tan tien). Breathing also allows us to feel. One reason we hold our breath is to avoid feeling or crying. Thinking can block feeling.

Practitioners must breathe along with their clients. Long, slow, deep breaths using the diaphragm. The diaphragm drops on the inhale and the pelvic floor naturally moves up to assist on the exhale. Coach your client to breathe this way. Assist them by putting a small amount of pressure with your flat hand against their lower abdomen, just above the pubic bone. This will give them something to push against on the inhale. The belly will rise up and expand on the inhale, allowing the lungs to fill completely. Don't rush the breath, but encourage a full breath and a complete exhale.

The breath represents inspiration and respiration; re-spiriting the body or spiritualizing matter.

Breathing oxygenates and alkalinizes the blood, taking us away from a stress response. Acidic blood is not a healthy environment for our tissues.

As you are coaching your client with breathing you may see physical movement patterns reveal themselves in the body. Is the chest opening, are the shoulders moving, is the back arching, are the ribs expanding? Is there an ease and fullness with the breath? Or is it forced, shallow and unnatural? This observation will give you much information about what is happening in the client's body. It is information that you may find useful later, but it may not be the focus of this particular treatment.

If your client's chest is very tight or the pectoral muscles are very strong you may assist your client on the exhale by pressing down on the sternum. This will allow them to exhale completely. The heart, lungs, lymph and all the internal organs benefit from a strong full breath. The large intestines are suspended at the flexures (splenic flexure and hepatic flexure) to the diaphragm. The heart rests on top of the diaphragm; a strong deep breath allows the heart to ride along. So enjoy a full breath.

If the ribs are glued down and not allowing a full breath we will loosen the tissues under the ribcage during our Chi Nei Tsang session. The opening of this space under the ribs is key to freeing up other organs like the stomach and liver.

Breathing may evoke an emotional insight or release. This may be as subtle as a slight energetic discharge, shudder, aha moment, etc. Or it could come as a release of tears and emotion. These moments are very important in the process of healing. The release of stuck energies and emotions brings the body into the present moment. We do not need to understand it or explain it, we only need to allow it to happen. As a Chi Nei Tsang therapist, you do not need to become a psycho-analyst. Ride it like a wave and it will naturally discharge and come to stillness and integration. The client is now ready to experience life from a fresh place. Think of it as spring cleaning for the cells. Emotions can weigh on the cells like a heavy blanket if they are not allowed motion.

Remember, it is the body that is processing life and digesting experiences and emotions – the belly is our second brain – so don't try to language the treatment. The body has its own language.

Working From the Navel

We begin Chi Nei Tsang treatments with connection to the breath, and move to working around the navel. Why is the navel so important? Why is it the simplest and most profound part of CNT treatments? This is the very first technique that Master Chia saw his teacher Mui Wattanaba use to treat his uncle's shoulder problem. It worked, and Master Chia was enthralled by this type of healing from the navel.

Embryologically our physical bodies grow from the navel and it is from this place that we source ourselves in the physical world. It begins with the Ovum. The first cell division creates the facial plane that we know as the Microcosmic Orbit, the next division creates the eight extraordinary vessels. At three weeks the embryo is a plate of cells made up of three layers that will differentiate into all the different systems in the body. By day 33 we can identify a mesentery that will become the organs. A portion of what will become the small intestine can be found in the umbilical cord. Later, as the tissues rotate the mesentery remains to suspend, support and separate the small intestines. The mesentery beneath the small intestine is a series of many layers and folds of overlapping fascia. The organs begin to migrate up and down, right and left, and the fascial planes fold over like a croissant.

The navel is the original location for the cellular and connective tissue development and migration of all the organs. The cells that eventually became our brain shared the same cellular origin and location as the enteric nervous system (small intestine), and later migrated to their location in the head. It is why we call the belly the second brain, and in fact, there is more information transmitted from the belly to the brain, than from the brain to the belly.

Our "gut feelings" are really messages from the abundant neuro-receptor sites in the gut.

During fetal development the cells fold and unfold, rotate and migrate like a living croissant. It is an elegant dance rather than a game of pin the tail on the donkey. It happens in the connective tissue (fascia) and the three dimensional fluid matrix, providing the architecture for our body to communicate as it stretches out to create meridians and organs.

Our original connection to the physical world remains as our navel. The umbilical cord nourished us and carried away waste during our time in the womb. The connective tissue inside the rim of the navel has a connection to our entire body. Working inside the navel can result in some of the most amazing results, such as a release of the spine, cessation of menstrual cramps, and musculoskeletal restrictions as far away as the fingers.

The shape of the navel can give you a clue into the deeper body tensions and the amount of chi that is available to this person. If the navel is pulled or twisted this indicates that there is a visceral pulling or twisting somewhere in the abdomen. 90% of musculoskeletal restrictions have a visceral component.

With palpation and visual inspection, you can follow the restrictions from the navel to other places in the body and unwind the connective tissues that have become stuck and dehydrated. This causes a slowing of neurological information that is trying to move through the fluid architecture of the fascia on its way to the brain, and creates pain as the dehydrated receptor cites get glued together, causing chronic pain sensations.

Working inside the upper half of the inner rim of the navel for 30 minutes or more is not unheard of. In fact, you could spend the entire treatment working at the navel. It is profound and simple.

Ideally the navel would be round and deep. This indicates the ability to store and hold chi throughout the day. A shallow navel or one that is sealed shut like the end of a balloon indicates a lack of life force, limited chi, and poor digestion. A navel with a twisted, spiraling shape may indicate a twist in the spine. The navel reveals many things about the body and the mesentery and organs beneath the navel itself.

Now that we have enlisted the breath and worked inside the rim of the navel, we can move our attention to the large intestine.

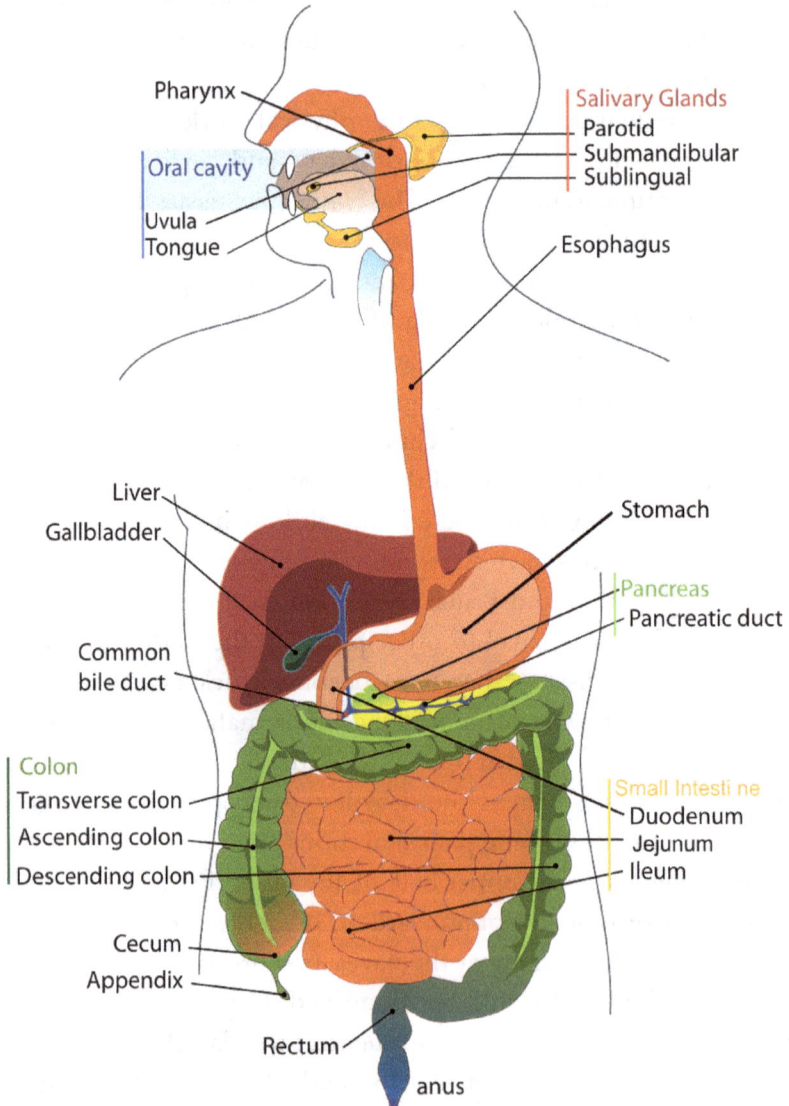

Introducing the Organs

The Large Intestine

Our digestive system is a long tube which begins at the mouth and ends at the anus. Even worms have a digestive system, they don't have a brain, but worms share our ability to digest. In fact, our digestive system is the oldest part of our bodies, our brains are the newer adaptations.

The large intestine receives waste via the ileocecal valve from the small intestine. After the small intestine has absorbed the last bit of nutrients from the food we have eaten, it empties into the cecum. On the lower right side of the abdomen you will find the ascending colon, the cecum and the appendix. This area can be tender and if it is compromised with adhesions from surgery or injury the ileocecal valve may have trouble opening and closing normally. If it is jarred open the toxic contents of the large intestine may flow backwards, possibly causing headaches and diarrhea, or become a breeding ground for parasites. You will learn to palpate this area in class.

Everything in the belly and pelvis is held by suspensory ligaments and connective tissues. Some women have extra tight suspensory ligaments in the lower right side of the pelvis, possibly from the cecum to the right ovary. Tight ligaments can pinch down onto nerves that are trying to pass through the obturator foramen on the way to the leg. If these nerves are pinched a person may experience unexplained knee pain. Freeing up the area with Chi Nei Tsang and creating more space and fluidity can bring relief from nagging pain in the leg and knee. Focused abdominal massage does allow connective tissue to melt and move.

The ascending colon makes a turn at the hepatic flexure. More like a fold, it changes direction and begins its transit from the right lower rib cage across the body to the left flexure, the splenic flexure. You will not be able to easily palpate the transverse colon as it is deep, but you will be able to create more space as you stretch the tissues down from under the rib cage, relaxing the diaphragm

The descending colon moves down the left side of the abdomen before making a gentle curve into the sigmoid colon and then emptying in the rectum. It is in this final stretch of descending colon that the waste can become dry. One of the jobs of the large intestine is to keep an electrolyte and water balance in the body by drawing out any excess fluid that is in the large intestine. Therefore, if waste stays in this part of the large intestine too long you can become constipated. Chi Nei Tsang is particularly helpful in creating movement and fluidity here. And it is precisely in this area that we begin to clear the large intestine.

Chi Nei Tsang treatments massage the descending colon, the transverse colon, and lastly the ascending colon. Repeating this pattern several times is very beneficial to elimination. Cats Paws, a rock and pump movement, is especially helpful to create fluidity and relaxation in the abdomen, followed by specific gentle movements with your fingers to find areas that are congested and creating external stimulation of the large intestine assisted by the breathing and internal movement from the client.

Probiotics keep the large intestine healthy, as do fermented foods. The probiotics that we ingest do not populate the gut, but rather carry away toxins, especially heavy metals. So, we need to eat them every day. Antibiotics wipe out beneficial bacteria. Antidepressants and opiate drugs freeze the neuro-receptor sites in the gut causing more numbing and constipation. There are more receptor sites in the gut than in the brain.

95% of the body's Serotonin is produced in the intestines. Serotonin changes the motility of your bowels (how fast food moves through), affects how much fluid, like healthy mucous, is secreted in your intestines, and affects how sensitive your intestines are to sensations like pain and fullness. Overall, serotonin is very important to our ability to rest and digest. Serotonin is considered a natural mood stabilizer. It's the chemical that helps with sleeping, eating, and digesting.

Serotonin also helps:

- reduce depression
- regulate anxiety
- heal wounds
- maintain bone health
- changes the motility of your bowels
- affects how much fluid is secreted in your intestines
- affects how sensitive your intestines are to sensations like pain and fullness

The large intestine does not digest foods, so if the stomach and small intestine have not been able to break down all the proteins, which is a lack of digestive fire, then a person may experience gas and farting as the undigested proteins move through the large intestine.

Colon health is connected to Bone health. The colon is largely responsible for water absorption and the absorption of vitamins that the gut flora produces (vitamin K, vitamin B12, thiamine, riboflavin)

Important micronutrients in bones are calcium, phosphorous, fluoride, magnesium, sodium, vitamin D, vitamin A, vitamin C, vi-tamin B6, folate, and vitamin B12. Vitamin K1 (from leafy green vegetables) is what we normally hear about (usually vitamin K is mentioned in relation to proper blood clotting). But vitamin K2 (produced by our gut flora) travels to the bone tissue and helps activate osteoblasts.

While most calcium and magnesium is absorbed by the small intestine, when absorption in the small intestine is compromised, the large intestine can increase its absorption of these and other vital minerals.

A healthy colon proves to be important for bones. Those individuals with inflammatory bowel disease (like Crohn's and Ulcerative Colitis) commonly also have osteoporosis, and these individuals also tend to have a poor microbiome.

Positive emotions associated with the large intestine (paired organ with the lungs) include: having the courage to feel one's feelings and the discernment and maturity to let go of what is no longer needed. Negative emotions associated with the large intestine (paired organ with the lungs) include: grief, sadness and depression.

The Liver

There is so much to say about the liver, our health is critically dependent on a healthy liver. It metabolizes carbohydrates, fats, lipids, proteins, drugs, hormones, toxins and vitamins. The liver pumps three pints of blood per minute. It stores and filters blood, nutrients and toxins. More than 500 functions have been attributed to the liver. Nutrients from our food travel via the portal vein directly from the small intestine into the liver for distribution. There are priorities, of course. And one of them is to handle toxins on a daily basis. Therefore the liver is active at night, when we are naturally sleeping, between 11pm and 3am. Good sleep is a pre requisite to good health. Toxins are sent out to be eliminated from the body, or shuttled away from the organs to protect them, and stored in fat.

Bacterial toxins enter the bloodstream and end up in the liver, yet these toxins can exceed the liver's detoxifying capacity. Toxic waste then migrates into the body and causes painful symptoms. The liver does the cleaning, but it does not take out the trash. That job is the responsibility of other organs in the body and other processes which are a part of several detox pathways.

One quart of bile is produced every day to emulsify fats that we eat. Bile also carries away bacteria and other toxins. We need to eat a minimum of two tablespoons of healthy fat every day to stimulate the gallbladder to release bile. Ideally, we eat a substantial lunch and empty the gallbladder each day so that bile does not condense into stones.

The liver can regenerate in six weeks, which is why liver surgery and replacement is possible. Our body is constantly regenerating and replacing itself with new cells. We are 90% new every year.

In Chinese medicine we say that cancers and tumors are created by fire toxins. This would indicate that the liver cannot keep up with the demands we are putting on it by our lifestyle and food choices.

Symptoms of liver stagnation:

- Weight gain around the abdomen
- Cellulite
- Abdominal bloating
- Indigestion
- High blood pressure
- Elevated cholesterol
- Fatigue
- Mood swings
- Depression
- Skin rashes

Liver Stressors:

- Caffeine
- Sugar
- Trans fats
- Medications
- Inadequate fiber
- Too much thinking and sitting
- Frustration

Positive emotions associated with the Liver (paired organ with the Gallbladder) include: clear thinking, patience, generosity, an ability to grow and change.

Negative emotions associated with the Liver (paired organ with the Gallbladder) include: frustration, impatience, anger, greed.

Detoxification Medicine

Detoxification Medicine is an ancient concept that appears as part of many healthcare systems around the world and is offered at my health spas.

There are three areas of concern in the physical realm:

1. heavy metal exposure
2. pesticides and solvents
3. intestinal ecology

The main organs of detoxification are the liver, large intestine and kidneys. Lungs and skin are also important, as we breathe and sweat out some toxins. We directly address all of these in our CNT treatments.

There are also emotional toxins, our thoughts and emotions can create a toxic environment for our cells. Both physical and emotional toxins affect the metabolism of the organs and one's overall sense of well-being. Chi Nei Tsang and traditional Chinese medicine address both physical and emotional toxins, offering healing with massage, qigong and meditations. Chi Nei Tsang treatments may assist the body to detox, and treatments are a perfect adjunct to a detox program.

There are six detox pathways. The body is designed to have multiple ways to stay healthy. Not everyone has all six available to them, however, so if you are eating broccoli and soaking in sulfur springs but feeling worse, you may have a genetic inability to detox sulfur. Genetic testing and the support of a Naturopath would be a good choice.

Also, the body has to be warm enough to detox; the liver and thyroid work together on this. Eating cold greens is not a good choice in keeping the liver and small intestine warm and functional. Warm, far intra red mats have been used recently to assist in detox when the body is burdened with excess toxins. Many cultures used under the floor heating and sleeping shelves to stay healthy in winter. Traditionally, planning to detox in the spring and sum-mer when the weather is warm supports the body's natural rhythm and function.

Here are six classic steps to detox that I discuss in the Spring Rejuvenation and Longevity retreat:

1. Remove the obstacles to health (our addictions)
2. Improve circulation
3. Enhance elimination
4. Repair the gastrointestinal system
5. Stimulate the liver
6. Transform Stress

This is classic detox medicine that points to the efficacy of Chi Nei Tsang treatments in assisting the body both physically and emotionally. The hands-on treatment speeds up the metabolism by moving in more chi and by creating movement, therefore speeding the movement of toxins from the body. The six healing sounds supports the cooling and re-balancing of the organ's emotional chi, transforming stress. Chi Nei Tsang treatments definitely help with elimination and circulation of blood and lymph.

Detoxing is not a pleasant experience and we often avoid it. Typical symptoms are headache, nausea, fatigue, inability to think clearly, aches and pains, skin eruptions, and poor sleep. Once we begin to detox it is critical that we drink enough water to keep the uncovered toxin moving out of the body. Lemon juices support phases one and two of detox. Glutathione, an enzyme found in fresh fruits and vegetables, is required as a phase one catalyst, and also conjugates toxins in phase two to escort them from the body.

A complete detoxification therapy should include:

- dietary therapy to heal the intestinal flora
- nutritional supplements
- sauna therapy to reduce fat stored pesticides.

Once you detox, be mindful of the retox!

Small Intestine

The small intestine is our second brain, and home to our digestive fire. In order to have good health we need to manifest the digestive fire inside of us. The small intestine is our fire element; 15 feet of potent organ chi designed to extract nutrients from our food, transforming what we ingest into something that will support our physicality. The small intestine separates the pure from the impure. Digestion is also the process of elimination. 90% of the absorption of nutrients happens here and is sent via the portal vein to the liver for distribution. Transformation happens with heat; eating warm cooked foods. Fire in nature transforms one substance to another and leaves a residue of waste behind. The small intestine grasps the nutrients in foods and destroys toxins in the gut. If it is weak it cannot digest and assimilate nutrients, and toxins increase. Cold foods, raw foods and unripe fruits are more difficult to digest, and can cool the gut and cause cramping. If the fire in the gut is too low use warming, spicy, and aromatic foods.

The small intestine is called the second brain, when in fact, there are more neurotransmitters here in the gut than in our brains, and more information is being sent from the gut to the brain than the other direction. Heard the expression "gut feeling"? The new saying is mood/food. There are more neurons in the intestines that in the entire spinal column. They enable independent perception, learning, memory and behavior; direct life experience. In CNT we say that the gut digests our life experiences.

There is a cleansing wave in the small intestine that happens in 90-minute intervals when we are not eating. It is meant to move out excess and roughage. Too much roughage may lead to symptoms of small intestinal bacterial overgrowth (SIBO). It is a good idea to abstain from eating for 3-5 hours between meals in order for the small intestine to complete it's cleansing wave. The ileocecal valve at the juncture between small intestine and ascending colon is designed to prevent bacteria that belong in the colon from moving backward into the small intestine. Chi Nei Tsang treatments are often effective in stimulating this valve to respond normally.

There are approximately 600 types of bacteria in the gut, of which we have identified about 20%. Balance is key, and when we are out of balance, we experience symptoms that can lead to leaky gut, diverticulitis, and SIBO, (small intestinal bacterial overgrowth). Many people with these symptoms or diagnoses have a recent history of food poisoning which interrupted the gut microbiome. This can happen anytime, especially during traveling. The lining of the intestine can become irritated and swollen which interferes with the proper messages of hunger and satiation.

The mesenteric root of the small intestine can limit mobility in the spine as it connects to the third and fourth lumbar vertebrae. Scars in the belly from surgery or infection can pull on vertebrae and cause restricted motion. Organs which are blocked from normal movement can interfere with nerves and joints, causing hard to explain symptoms. It is thought that up to 90% of musculoskeletal problems have a visceral component. Chi Nei Tsang treatments can bring much welcome relief from deep restrictions and limited range of motion.

The progression of disease that can occur in the intestines often involves an emotional component. In fact, our emotions can be the cause of many symptoms and so, both the physical and the emotional needs to restore health must be addressed

Positive emotions associated with the small intestine (paired organ with the heart): joy, inspiration, compassion, enthusiasm for life

Negative emotions associated with the small intestine (paired organ with the heart): rage, judgement, hatred

Leaky Gut

The lining of your gut is like a net with tiny holes in it that only allow specific molecules to pass through into the blood stream. The gut lining is a barrier to keep out bigger particles that can damage your body. If the lining of your gut is damaged the net loses its integrity, so proteins like gluten, bad bacteria, undigested food, and toxins leak from inside your intestinal wall into your blood stream. This may cause an immune reaction and if it continues may lead to autoimmune conditions.

The inflammation that leaky gut causes creates symptoms such as bloating, food sensitivities, fatigue, thyroid conditions, joint pain, headaches, digestive problems, weight gain, crohns, diver-ticulitis and IBS. Science is also recognizing the link between gut health and mental health; mood and food.

The causes of leaking gut may include poor diet, chronic stress, an overload of toxins and bacterial overgrowth. Lectins play a large part in causing the irritation and subsequent tissue swelling that people with SIBO experience. Lectins are proteins found in grains including wheat, rice, soy, legumes (like cashews).

To begin healing this sensitivity one must remove foods and other factors (like stress) that damage the gut. Rebalance the gut with probiotics. Yes, take them every day as many probiotics carry out toxins. Fermented foods are a must in your diet, get some variety. Many probiotics do not populate in the gut, they are just passing through which is why we need to eat them daily. Foods to support gut health are Bone broth (make it yourself), Goat milk kefir, fermented vegetables, (also easy to make at home) coconut products, omega 3's, lamb and salmon.

Irritable Bowel Syndrome
(IBS and SIBO)

At this time the diagnosis of SIBO (small intestinal bacterial overgrowth) seems to be on the rise, and the treatment options are not always successful. Gut bacteria are out of balance and responding, or not responding to foods and antibiotics. Bacteria are one of the oldest living life forms on earth and there are more bacteria cells in the human body than there are human cells. 300-600 different types of bacteria have been found in the gut. Scientists have, so far, cultured about 20%, the rest are unknown to us. And each of us has our own bacterial fingerprint that develops when we are young.

Clients with irritable bowel syndrome and SIBO do experience relief from Chi Nei Tsang treatments. Often they feel full and hungry at the same time because the inner lining of the bowel is swollen. This swelling response happens most often from food allergies, or from foods that create more of an imbalance in gut bacteria. Healing is possible, but takes time and diligence to avoid setbacks. You can feel this swollen tissue with your touch as you give a CNT treatment. Gentle touch will help to release some of the swelling. Another symptom is a binding or knotting in random parts of the large intestine. It is not understood why this happens, but many people suffer with this symptom. The intestine clamps down on itself, and blocks the movement of peristalsis. Gentle massage is helpful.

Stomach and Duodenum

Most of us are aware of our stomachs on an hourly basis. Empty, hungry? Full and Satisfied? Too full? Achy, nauseas, tense. Endless feelings on both sides of the spectrum from good to bad. The stomach, being our Earth element in Chinese Medicine, can bring us to a place of balance and a sense of abundance and practicality. Emotions typically guide our thinking and eventually inform our actions and behaviors. This defines our personality. There are many other emotions associated with the stomach which come from body image and the choice to starve our bodies in order to look good. This creates a deep division in our body-mind and confuses our ability to feel well and self-satisfied.

A muscular tube, the stomach is surrounded by nerves that branch out from the vagus nerve. Muscular and smooth on the outside, acidic and ridged with gastric folds on the inside. The epithelial cells inside the stomach create an acidic environment meant to break down proteins. This is where the heavy lifting begins, after we have chewed our food. Food then passes through the pyloric sphincter into the duodenum where it is mixed with bile and alkaline enzymes from the pancreas into a perfect digestive mix. This mix is sent on to the small intestine to finish the alchemical process of extraction of nutrients.

If the stomach is not creating enough acid, which happens as we age, or as a result of our diet, then we can assist protein breakdown by drinking a teaspoon of apple cider vinegar with meals. This gives the stomach a boost, rather than taking over its function like other digestive aids do. Undigested food down the line will cause gas and bloating.

A part of the Earth element, the pancreas is an endocrine gland and also a digestive organ. Eating too much sugar can create a hardening of the pancreas. The spleen is often referred to in Earth element, but it is actually a lymph node which breaks down bacteria, not a digestive organ. It stores and filters blood, about 1 ½ pints. My feeling is that the meridian associated with spleen is actually moving toward the pancreas.

Positive emotions associated with the Stomach (paired organ with the Pancreas) include: satisfaction, practicality, support, abundance, balance

Negative emotions associated with the Stomach (paired organ with the Pancreas) include: anxiety, worry, out of balance,

Kidneys

The kidneys are deep, retroperitoneal, and protected. Fragile and Yin, they filter fluids and regulate the minerals and pH. balance of the body. The kidneys also eliminate toxins that are moved out from the liver.

During our development in utero the kidneys shared some of the same tissue as our sexual organs, and therefore, in Chinese Medicine you will see reference to the kidneys, sexual energy, and ancestral energy.

We will not be able to palpate the kidneys, but we can work energetically to sense and feel the health and vitality of them. One indication of a problem is stinky feet. Why? The kidneys eliminate waste through the bladder, but excess waste via lymph may be passing through the interstitial tissues of the legs along the kidney meridian to the bottoms of the feet.

We will look at how to work with the kidneys from a side lying position and apply this technique to other situations such as preg-nancy.

Positive emotions associated with the Kidneys (paired organ with the Bladder) include: trust, gentleness, ability to be in flow

Negative emotions associated with the Kidneys (paired organ with the Bladder) include: fear, mistrust, forcing of one's will.

Other Body Systems Involved In Treatment

The Fascia

Every organ, muscle, nerve and bone are surrounded, supported and protected by a layer of fascia – connective tissue. The folding and overlapping of many fascial planes during embryological development of the fetus explains the connection between organs and the diversity of meridians used in Chinese Medicine.

Fascia and connective tissue interconnects the entire body and is found in every cell in the body. Fascia is denser around the heart and kidneys and more loosely woven on the face. There are many layers of fascia in the body.

The visceral layers surround and connect the organs. In fact, the organs communicate via vibration and the position of the connective tissues. Fascia in the brain moves downward to become the sheath of the spinal cord and outward to the nerves. With every breath we take (24,000 times a day), the diaphragm is moving up and down on the organs and the pelvic floor, giving and receiving information. The fascia is sending bioelectric signals between every part of the body. Indeed, connective tissue is the most abundant tissue in the body. This three dimensional fluid matrix supports, protects and stabilizes every part of your body.

Due to the nature of fascia, there is a continuous flow of information along the connective tissue, and therefore we are able to touch the navel and affect the big toe or the ear at the same time. Tom Myers, in his book Anatomy Trains, explains fascial lines in the body, saying that there is a relationship between the fascia and the autonomic nervous system; many ganglia are found embedded in fascial planes. There are numerous sensory nerve endings in connective tissues which send pain messages to the brain and communicate information to other parts of the body.

Embryologically, the paired organs evolved from the same tissues and migrated to their natural positions. The meridians described in Chinese medicine pass from superficial to deep fascia in the organs. The mesentery of the gut is sourced from the same tissues as the heart. This is the basis of the heart and small intestine relationship to the fire element. For a time during development there is communication between the brain tissues and the gut tissues. Indeed, science now tells us that there are more messages sent from the gut to the brain than from brain to belly. The research of Taro Kashio M.D. has demonstrated that there is a strong relationship between a blockage in the descending colon and cerebral hemorrhages in the left hemisphere.

Light pressure and massage, such as CNT, will affect the position and function of the organs as the fascia becomes more fluid and information is allowed to flow in the body. Where there is stuck stress or dehydration in connective tissues from posture, injury, surgery, or infection, the information is not flowing and there is often chronic pain.

Chi Nei Tsang treatments can bring fluidity and rehydration to these tissues which allow organs to communicate again without blockage. This in turn relieves pain and improves metabolism. The key is to work gently and slowly. Too much pressure will trigger the pain signal in the fascia.

"Be sure that you apply pressure gently with the flat part of your hand and the flat parts of your fingertips. Do not poke with the tips of your fingers as this can be a very sensitive region on people. If a client has a very tight abdomen, do not force the muscles to move by adding pressure. Be patient and keep applying light pressure and some clients will release their muscle tension. This does not always happen, so do not force it by any means." (Mochizuki)

The Lymph System

The Lymph collects bacteria, toxins, metabolic by products, inert matter, and other cellular debris from tissues everywhere in the body, via extracellular fluid, and transports these waste products to various sites of elimination. Within the large lymphatic junctions known as lymph nodes antibodies and white blood cells are produced. Lymph nodes are a pre filter before the blood is sent to the liver.

There is more lymph than blood in the body; about 15 liters, three times the amount of blood. The lymphatic system is part of the body's immune system and consists of a network of approximately 600-700 fluid filled sacs and vessels distributed throughout the entire body just under the surface of the skin and within the body cavity.

Chi Nei Tsang is a fantastic treatment to affect movement in the deep lymph of the belly and groin. The cisterna chyli which is deep near L1 and L2 (near the navel), is a large lymph sac that collects from the limbs and abdomen. Occasionally hardened lymph edema can be felt in the belly, and in the omentum.

A large portion of the lymphatic system resides inside the small intestines, where many small nodes (Peyer's patches) are embedded in the tissue of the intestinal walls. At least 60 percent of the immune system is hidden in these nodes, which constitute what is known as gut associate lymph tissue. GALT.

It appears that most of the body's immune screening system is located here to facilitate the screening of all food and the potentially harmful hitchhikers that can accompany that food before it enters the bloodstream. Most of our daily immune function is made up of the complex interaction between diet, intestinal bacteria and GALT.

GALT is also part of the communications network that links the intestines with the rest of the body, especially the brain.

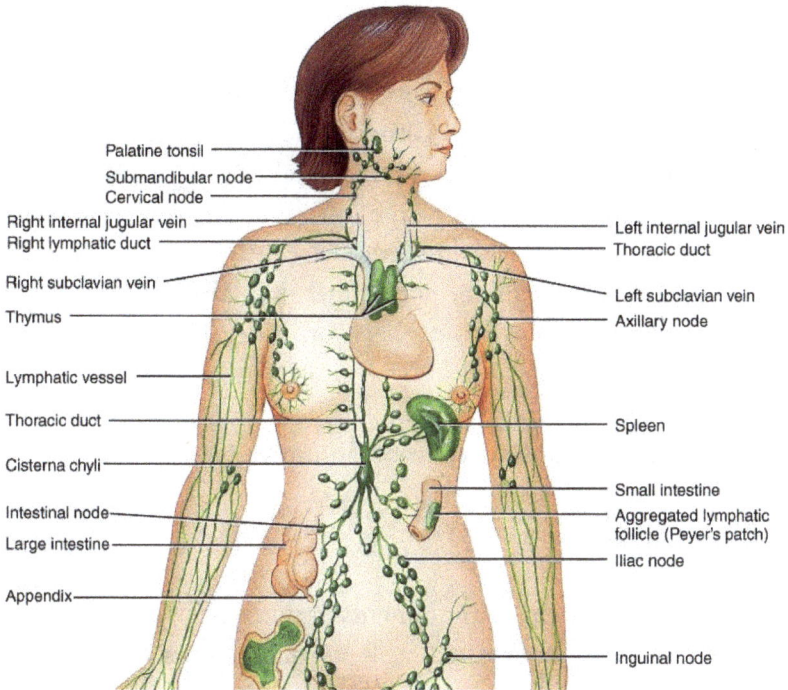

Palatine tonsil
Submandibular node
Cervical node
Right internal jugular vein
Right lymphatic duct
Right subclavian vein
Thymus
Lymphatic vessel
Thoracic duct
Cisterna chyli
Intestinal node
Large intestine
Appendix

Left internal jugular vein
Thoracic duct
Left subclavian vein
Axillary node
Spleen
Small intestine
Aggregated lymphatic follicle (Peyer's patch)
Iliac node
Inguinal node

Look at a picture of the lymph nodes near the large intestine, you may also see the messentary in the background that attaches to the large intestine. Find a good anatomical book, like a Netters Anatomy book.

The Omentum

The greater omentum develops from the mesentery (connective tissues) that connects the stomach to the posterior abdominal wall. It grows during fetal development to cover the majority of the small and large intestine. The omentum looks like an apron of bubble wrap that covers the organs and is found just below the surface of the abdominal skin. You may feel lumpy parts of the omentum as you work on the belly during a CNT treatment.

The functions of the greater omentum are:
1. Excess Fat storage
2. Immune cells in the form of "milky spots"

Most of the action in the omentum takes place in clusters of white blood cells, known officially as milky spots, that dot the organ. They serve as a kind of filter for the abdominal fluid that circulates through the omentum and play a role in controlling immune responses to bacteria in the gut.

3. Infection and wound isolation: The greater omentum can often be found wrapped around areas of infection and trauma

Chi Nei Tsang Treatment Overview

You have all taken a class in Chi Nei Tsang, or experienced a treatment. Much of this information is now a review and a reminder. No two treatments are ever the same.

What is a treatment like?

Clients lie on a massage table, or sometimes on the floor, on their backs, fully clothed, knees bent, belly exposed. The practitioner begins by placing their hands on the clients' abdomen and coaches the client to breathe into the belly, which directs awareness to the belly and therefore to the entire body/mind. The very act of breathing may illicit emotional release.

It is when we hold our breath that we block feeling and emotion. When we hold back our breathing we are often in fear, or thinking only with the mind.

Healing occurs when the client connects their breath and awareness of what is there in the belly, our second brain. Stepping outside of the thinking mind, the body connects to its deeper wisdom and healing occurs non-verbally. What you become aware of begins to change. This is a fact in Quantum physics; observation creates an event. I like to think of this process as the anchoring of life and essence. It is an anchoring of the breath of spirit into the dimension of life. Simple yet profound; which is the beauty of this ancient healing method. The breath becomes the metaphor for life; inhaling inspiration, exhaling and letting go of the past. Savoring the pause between breaths, the simple act of breathing becomes a way to measure one's life. Respiration is re-spiriting. As we breathe with awareness, we spiritualize matter.

One way to calm the body and the vagus nerve is through deep breathing. The vagus nerve comes from the brain and controls the parasympathetic nervous system, which controls your relaxation response. This nerve activates the organs throughout the body (such as the heart, lungs, liver and digestive organs).

Healthy vagal tone is indicated by a slight increase of heart rate when you inhale, and a decrease of heart rate when you exhale. Deep diaphragmatic breathing—with a long, slow exhale—is key to stimulating the vagus nerve and slowing heart rate and blood pressure. 80-90% of the nerve fibers in the vagus nerve are dedicated to communicating the state of your viscera to your brain. When people say "trust your gut" they are in many ways saying "trust your vagus nerve." Candace Pert wrote in Molecules of Emotion, that "emotions are felt throughout the body as sensations. Emotions consist of organic changes in the body, muscular and visceral."

Sessions may bring up strong emotions. Tears, body memories and emotions can come easily and move quickly away in a session bringing clients forward in time to a place of peace, ease, rest, joy. The dimensions traversed during a one-hour treatment are many. Clients quickly move into an altered state where time/space are one, not linear, not measured by a clock. That part of the brain that orients us in time and space goes quiet, so that the body may process and integrate quickly. As a practitioner I focus intently on holding the portals open for the client to travel beyond and back. Most cry and laugh and drop deeply into what only the body knows. What is touched softly by the hands can be described as essence and life.

Tensions held in the belly let go and the spine relaxes the effort of holding a compromised posture. Our physical posture often mirrors our emotional posture. Organs move into a new rhythm with each other allowing the symphony to harmonize. New life force moves through the cells to lift away toxic emotions and toxic chemicals. The organs experience new vitality and better function. Simple and Profound. The metabolism shifts, the structure shifts, the spirit settles into the body. Incarnation becomes a reality for the first time for many clients. The deep emotional charges that have been clogging the evolution of the being and the gross metabolism of the organs are released.

Words are not really necessary as the body processes our undigested emotional experiences. The proof is in the tasting of the pudding, as was said in the past, and the proof of the benefit of CNT is often seen immediately in a relief of symptoms, or a change in behavior or perspective (which is real healing for most people). I have witnessed people change jobs, relationships, and their daily patterns. I have seen people experience and feel themselves in new ways. Some are finally free of pain and grief which will stand in the way of forward progress. Our inner world becomes reflected into our outer world.

I felt after my first few CNT treatments a new experience of freedom and being truly in the present moment like never before. The past had fallen away and the energy in my body was available to me without the restrictions or burden of the past. I truly had no idea that I was carrying a burden around in my body.

Many people connect the physical body with the emotions that are held there. Sometimes these physical feelings and emotions are not comfortable, but on a deep gut level we know that it is necessary to feel this in order to move forward. I have spoken with several practitioners and clients who at first went through a healing transition as a result of CNT treatment. All the while knowing that this is what the body and spirit were craving. When there is no resistance we can move into our destiny.

The energetic/chi contact is deep. Clients move into a deeply relaxed state during CNT treatments, time and space are altered, relaxation is profound. Most clients feel that they have been sleeping, although remaining acutely aware of everything. It is a fact that when we shift brain waves to theta, where most healing happens quickly, our brain loses track of time and space, as supported by a study at Columbia University on brain waves and meditation.

Anchoring the Lower Tan Tien

The Lower Tan Tien is an energetic location in the belly be-low the navel. Also called the Sea of Chi, and the Cauldron in Taoist practices, this area connects the body to a deeper level of physical manifestation via the central channel. We could say that the belly is between heaven and Earth, at the level of humanity. Chi flows from heaven through the organs toward Earth, bring-ing spiritual information about our incarnation. Chi flows upward from Earth through the organs towards heaven bringing evolu-tionary information about our bodies. Any blockage in the organs slows down the transmission of information and also hampers our body's metabolism.

The Lower Tan Tien also stores Jing, raw physical energy, which interacts with chi and shen; breath and spirit. These three treasures, Jing Chi and Shen, become balanced with meditations such as the Microcosmic Orbit meditation and Qigong practices.

I use my elbow to anchor the Lower Tan Tien during CNT treatments. The elbow is a broader surface then a finger, and I am able to sink slowly and deeply over a long period of time without causing pain to my hands or to the client's belly. When I feel my elbow contact a warm fluid energy, I know that I have contacted the sea of chi and I stay at this position for a couple minutes, not sinking deeper or moving up, but staying connected to the client's breath. The sensation of being anchored into one's central chan-nel is relaxing and comforting on a body and spirit level. When we tap into these dimensions clients often drop into a slightly altered state of consciousness. My opinion is that if we are not anchored fully into our central channel, which is the level of our incarna-tion, then it can be difficult for the body to be at ease and heal.

I always do this technique in a CNT treatment to connect the body to its deeper level of intention for healing.

The Wind Gates

A wind gate is a portal, like an acupuncture point is a portal for chi to move in and out. Wind is translated as Chi. So opening a wind gate releases wind, or excess chi, or an accumulated charge in the body which may cause painful symptoms. We have an internal climate that is created by posture, food, emotions, overall health, etc. That internal climate creates a weather pattern in our body, like the weather we experience outside each day. Some days the weather is mild and pleasant, other days it is extreme and unpleasant. Winds that are too hot or too cold, or in excess, can create symptoms which lead to disease, and also cause structural pain.

There are eight wind gates located near the navel at the front of the belly. Four wind gates in the cardinal directions and four in diagonal directions. The first wind gate is to the left side of the navel, about a finger width away from the rim of the navel. We will be using our elbows to sink slowing into the wind gates, like we do when opening the Lower Tan Tien.

The wind gates are a mystery, so I hope you are okay with mysteries and things that cannot be explained. I have found that there is no exact reflexology map to the eight wind gates, however, the experience is real and profound for the client. You may sense hot or cold winds, winds that feel heavy or have some texture. Don't try to explain this, but do notice where in the body the client is feeling a connection. Chasing the winds from the belly and the rest of the body, too, is a large focus of the Chi Nei Tsang level two curriculum.

I open the wind gates at the beginning of a treatment to release excess pressure in the belly, and at the end of a treatment to bring everything back into balance. As with many aspects of Chi Nei Tsang treatments, this technique could become a major part and focus of any treatment.

Never force a wind gate to open, be patient and wait. If the gate does not open move on to the next wind gate.

This is a technique that needs to be learned from an instructor, and should also be experienced in your own body before trying to work on clients.

What To Do After A Session

My clients ask for feedback. Of course the best feedback is to feel and trust your own body. I may give them some simple advice or homework. Yes, that is right, homework. The session doesn't end when they slide off of the table with a smile or a look of surprise on their faces. Clients can continue self-care with the Six Healing Sounds and Inner Smile Meditations, bone breathing, working with the elements, Qigong, sleeping meditations, changing their diet, working on their own navel between sessions, and more. Ways to take self responsibility for healing are offered; simple guidance to steer clients back onto an easy path toward deeper and lasting healing.

Why Does This Work?

The body is very wise and responds quickly to Chi Nei Tsang treatments. Touch and breath are the first signals to enliven our physiology after we are born. The breath is the way in. When we breathe we quiet the mind. When we breathe we move out of fear and into the emotions. Healing begins by breathing into the belly. This is the unconditional support of Earth element that a practitioner can embody during sessions.

All of this occurs simultaneously while the hands move gracefully over the belly activating points in the body that release sound frequencies which metabolize emotional issues.

Emotions and Desires

Taoist and Buddhist monks and healers realized that our emotions, some of them being of low vibrations, create suffering and disease, and hold us in the earth plane and bring us back for lifetimes of clearing. Taoist meditations, in conjunction with CNT treatments work alchemically to clear the emotional body, freeing our energies for higher spiritual practices.

Meditation practice in feeling, understanding and directing primordial chi, or the light body, is one benefit of the Taoist foundation practices. Feeling is a key aspect. Taoist meditation is not about clearing the mind, but enlisting the mind to direct chi for healing, the goal being a felt sense of ease. Chi is intelligent information and can be directed for our healing process. Once the chi is moving, the mind can be quiet and contemplative. The Inner Smile and Six healing sounds meditation is an excellent example of an Alchemical Taoist meditation practice, which shifts unhealthy emotions that will block our organs health, into higher vibrations which are healthy and produce beneficial behaviors and actions.

Using the oldest archetypes of healing with sound and color, the organs and cells of the body respond as sound breaks up energetic patterns of stagnation and patterns of disease. Colors tone the cells of the body and the organs. Simple, yet profound. During a treatment, the practitioner may use the sound of the ocean waves breaking, Chooooooooo, to break up congestion in the kidneys, or project the color of a deep-sea blue/black into the kidneys to tonify them.

At the time of conception and even after birth babies can be tethered in by light, but there is a critical time in which to come in fully and for the physiology to fire up to sustain and anchor one in life. CNT anchors the body magnetically to the earth's field by activating magnetic spots in the belly (Lower Tan Tien or Sea of Chi), and releasing stagnant winds in the belly and other parts of the anatomy. We identify these points as the wind gates. CNT also stimulates the body's electrical system as happens after birth, stabilizing the physiology.

It is no wonder that many people live most of their lives with a feeling of not being at home here. In my work I have seen that many people are not grounded and have numerous difficulties as a result of this ranging from poor decision making to the manifestation of physical diseases. With so many humans on the planet feeling out of body and not at home, it begs the question, is the Earth a safe place? Einstein was once asked what he thought was the most important question of all time. He answered, "Is the Universe a safe place?" CNT creates safety for the body and it smooths over emotional release by aligning with the universal theme of "life supports you". One may then begin to perfect life and essence.

A good CNT practitioner allows time for the emotional body to clear and resettle. Since the monks did not give birth as such, they did master the art of getting each other fully into the body. CNT requires the focus and patience of a monk, or a good midwife. Birthing well requires purity of the heart and compassion, another attribute of a good healer. This purity is then imprinted, melted, into matter. As we clear daily emotions, we re-imprint upon our cells the purity we were conceived to express.

An advanced practitioner embodies compassion, joy, goodwill and detach-ment.

Using the archetypes of pulse and matter, the CNT practitioner vibrates the body into higher levels and the body spins off toxins. Many clients will experience a detoxifying response after treat-ment. Spirit pulses into the body and anchors along the magnetic grids. Later the body is purified with a high vibration of matter and pulse. Picture the image of water sliding over a rock. Water is the most powerful element, yet the most yielding and gentle. Water, as an element of creation will resonate sound and detoxify the body. Water creates electricity and charge. The connective tissue in every cell in your body is 80% water.

Just a side note, CNT is not a resonating model of healing as such, the healer does not resonate a frequency, but uses specific sounds to vibrate through the organs. For example, some healers will resonate a frequency from their Hara dimension; the dimension of incarnation and intention. Multi-faceted healers may be doing several things at once and resonating from other modalities, but this is not classical CNT.

How does a CNT healer sense the connection? The healer must breathe and there is often a mirroring of the client's breath that informs the healer what may be occurring inside of the client's body. When the client is connecting the breath to the belly the practitioner will feel movement or lack of movement, change in the tissues, notice temperature changes, see the skin and body change under their hands. The healer may witness a calming sensation in the body as it moves through the phases of connecting and letting go into quickly processing the mystery of healing and the fire of transformation. The integration may come swiftly or over time, as each of us has our own rhythm. The healer maintains contact with the whole person with the state of consciousness that nothing needs healing. The breath brings awareness, and once awareness comes healing cannot be avoided for long.

There are few preconditions for those who wish to practice this form of healing. Self-healing is always the first step. Training is open to anyone of any age. The practitioner must tap into their sea of chi in order to transmit it to others. A gentle safe touch is the only other requirement; soft hands, patience, compassionate understanding of the process of healing. As practitioners, we get out of the way and try not to fix anything. The message in the hands is that we are feeling a whole being who we honor and support in re balancing toward health.

What aspects and issues of the client are affected? Clients are affected physically, emotionally and spiritually, and thus the entire being is affected through all time and space. The template of the client's life and essence is cleared and evolved in the present, affecting the past and the future. In particular, the kidneys will hold one's ancestral issues. Generational issues tend to become concentrated in the kidneys. Our essential life energies, and specifically our sexual chi, is stored in the kidneys. Therefore, work in these organs may unwind generations of family wounding, allow for more ease during the birthing process, and assist the dying.

Working with the Elderly and Those with Advanced Diseases

Our focus for a healing session needs to be positive, hopeful, encouraging, educational, compassionate and realistic. There are times when our best efforts will bring a client into a state of peace and comfort, but will not eliminate a disease process. In these moments we must do our best to be present and honest with ourselves and the clients we serve. Quality of life is what most people want at the end of life, as well as deep contact with other humans. Real contact does not back away from the truth. Therefore, as a practitioner do your best to be knowledgeable and present with clients. Always be willing to put your hands on a person who asks for this type of healing intervention. A gentle touch is the most human and natural thing in the world.

Death and Dying

Chi Nei Tsang is an appropriate treatment modality to use when assisting those who are preparing to cross over. As the energies in the physical body begin to move upward and spiral outward, they are often stuck in the belly. The organs over time have become hardened and weak, slowing down the flow of chi. CNT treatments will bring more circulation and softening to the belly allowing for the chi to be directed up and out the crown of the head. In fact, most Taoist meditation is a preparation for a moment of conscious dying. Learning to keep a clear flow of chi circulating through one's microcosmic orbit and up the central channel to-ward the crown of the head is a fundamental meditation practice.

From a Taoist perspective, we incarnate through the central channel and anchor in the Lower Tan Tien. Anchoring the Lower Tan Tien is a very potent technique in a CNT treatment. When we are ready to exit, our chi moves back up through the central chan-nel toward the top of the head. Therefore, you are not going to anchor the tan tien of a dying person. You will also notice that the navel collapses, closes, and withdraws.

Chi Nei Tsang can be offered as a potent treatment anywhere on the planet. This is my firsthand experience. Just as we are born and die anywhere on this planet, the same can be said about the ability of CNT to heal us anywhere on the planet. Of course, working within a strong chi field will assist a practitioner with this work. Natural settings are the best.

An informed practitioner will be able to assist you from a dis-tance using the basic information of healing with sound and color, Qigong, food and lifestyle. I have tried incorporating the manual methods of CNT during a long-distance healing with some suc-cess, but I believe an in-person, hands on treatment is the best for this type of healing.

Chi Nei Tsang is simple and profound; it is truly an example of extraordinary healing. The evolution of our bodies' organs is tied to the evolution of the elements and the creation energies of the planet.

Chi Nei Tsang 1

Treatment Maps

The following treatment plans are meant to compliment your life training in a Chi Nei Tsang level 1 class. If you have taken this class with me, you will know that during trainings, at the end we touch upon how to craft a seamless treatment, summarizing what you have learned. Of course, what is presented here are only a few of the possible treatment scenarios that you will encounter. The following are based upon the standard model of a one-hour treatment. You may design your time with clients to include 10-15 minutes before and after in order to do an intake, and to allow for time to process and integrate what they experienced. I always schedule plenty of time between clients in my office so that they are not rushed, and so that I also can take care of myself. Please contact me at *whitecloudnm@aol.com* with any "what ifs" that may present themselves to you.

"An Ampuku session should last an average of 5-15 minutes (maximum 25 minutes)." Mochizuki. A Japanese Anma massage session would be included in this 25 minute focus on the abdomen.

By now you have learned about the anatomy and physiology of the organs, their association with the five elements, connective tissues and basic palpation skills. In your treatment approach, follow a Medical Qigong model of purge, tonify, balance. Purge toxins with sound, tonify with color, and balance Jing, Chi and Shen by harmonizing the breath and the belly. This type of treatment was called AnMo in Chinese Medicine for thousands of years.

Always use your informed intuition when you have your hands on a client and stay in the present moment with what arises.

Once these treatment suggestions are downloaded into your phone or computer, you can have them available to look at during a treatment. You may want to purchase a small projector to attach to your phone and project the treatment plan onto the wall. This will be very helpful when practicing the Advanced Chi Nei Tsang treatments which include points on the arms, legs, head and chest. In this way you can concentrate on being grounded, present and relaxed during your treatments.

The following treatment outlines provide the scaffolding for your treatments to blossom. Please connect your Chi field to the original energy signature and intention of this healing art. This was a potent healing practice before it was given a name. We are adapting this ancient healing art to our modern-day needs.

Basic 60 Minute CNT Introductory Treatment

1. Clear, ground and charge your Chi Field (1 minute)
2. Direct the client's breath into their belly (5 minutes)

Observe where the restrictions are, if any, in their breath.

3. Soften the belly with a kneading, back and forth, movement (5 minutes)

If the connective tissue is very tight, take more time to gently relax the tension and invite fluidity back into the tissues so that you can more easily palpate the organs.

4. Clear the large Intestine (10 minutes)
5. Soften the borders of the ribcage and pelvis (10 minutes)
6. Open the navel (10 minutes)

Observe shape and color.

7. Open the eight windgates (10 minutes)
8. Anchor the Lower Tan Tien (5 minutes)
9. Rest your hands on the belly, fill the organs with color (2 minutes)
10. Seal the client's Chi field and step away (2 minutes)

60 minutes

You may give the client a very brief overview of what you felt, if they ask. And give them some suggestions on how to take care of themselves at home, such as learning the six healing sounds, Qigong, etc.

You have heard me say many times that each part of a Chi Nei Tsang treatment (each technique) may be expanded to become the entire treatment. If a client needs help breathing, then focus on that. If a client is very constipated, then focus on that, etc.

As massage therapists we do not diagnose, however we can offer treatments that are specifically designed to assist clients at the place they need it the most. There are many reasons to work around the navel. I have witnessed many structural and spinal issues resolved with this treatment. Others have felt a release from the tension of menstrual pains. Since the small intestine and navel are embryologically linked we may see changes in digestion and metabolism. I offer this for you to explore.

Clearing and Opening of the Navel

1. Clear, ground and charge your Chi Field (1 minute)
2. Direct the client's breath into their belly (5 minutes)

   Observe where the restrictions are, if any, in their breath.
3. Soften the belly with a kneading, back and forth, movement (5 minutes)
4. Clear the large intestine (10 minutes)
5. Clear and open the navel (35 minutes)

   Observe the shape and color. When there is a lot of pink or red color around the navel it would indicate a release of heat and possibly toxins.

6. Rest your hands on the belly, fill the organs with color (2 minutes)
7. Seal the client's Chi field and step away (2 minutes)

60 minutes

Encourage your client to work on their own navel for a few minutes every day.

Working the fascia around and inside of the navel produces unique and unexpected results in the body. I have seen everything from relief of menstrual cramps to the unwinding of a whiplash neck injury. The vein that originally connected the umbilicus of the fetus to the liver during gestation has resolved into a band of tissue. There are numerous prenatal connections from the navel to the body. Working the navel is the most advanced, yet most simple of CNT treatments.

Detoxification Treatment

1. Clear, ground and charge your Chi Field (1 minute)
2. Direct the client's breath into their belly (5 minutes)

Observe where the restrictions are, if any, in their breath.

3. Soften the belly with a kneading, back and forth, movement (5 minutes)

If the connective tissue is very tight, take more time to gently relax the tension and invite fluidity back into the tissues so that you can more easily palpate the organs

4. Clear the large intestine (10 minutes)
5. Open the navel (10 minutes)
6. Soften the borders of the ribcage, opening space for liver (5 minutes)
7. Pump the liver. Rest your hands over the liver and send in the color green to tonify (15 minutes)
8. Anchor the Lower Tan Tien (5 minutes)
9. Rest your hands on the belly, fill the organs with color (2 minutes)
10. Seal the Client's Chi field and step away (2 minutes)

60 minutes

Detoxification has become an urgent issue for our bodies as we attempt to keep up with the new chemicals in our food and our environment. Remember that the major organs of detoxification are the lungs, large intestine, kidneys, liver and the skin. As I mentioned in class, Anchoring the Lower Tan Tien allows clients to be in their bodies fully in order to track what happens after CNT treatments. Urge clients to do more research if needed as this is a huge topic and deserves proper attention.

Digestive Issues

1. Clear, ground and charge your Chi Field (1 minute)
2. Direct the client's breath into their belly (5 minutes)

Observe where the restrictions are, if any, in their breath.
3. Soften the belly with a kneading, back and forth, movement (5 minutes)

If the connective tissue is very tight, take more time to gently relax the tension and invite fluidity back into the tissues so that you can more easily palpate the organs.

4. Clear the large intestine (10 minutes)
5. Soften the borders of the ribcage. Encourage the tissues which are stuck under the ribs back toward the navel. Create space for the stomach, pancreas and duodenum. Send in the color yellow, and make the sound, *Hoooooo*, to clear the Earth element (20 minutes)
6. Open the eight windgates (10 minutes)
7. Anchor the Lower Tan Tien (5 minutes)
8. Rest your hands on the belly, fill the organs with color (2 minutes)
9. Seal the client's Chi field and step away (2 minutes)

60 minutes

Digestive issues are complex and often include an overlay of emotions. There is not one diet that is good for everyone, so consulting with a Dietician may be of some benefit. If your client is having some emotional challenges please refer to part two of Gilles Marin's book, Five Elements, Six Conditions, for ideas on how to confront and change emotions that lead to disease.

Pelvic Health Treatment

1. Clear, ground and charge your Chi Field (1 minute)
2. Direct the client's breath into their belly (5 minutes)

Observe where the restrictions are, if any, in their breath.

3. Soften the belly with a kneading, back and forth, movement (5 minutes)

If the connective tissue is very tight, take more time to gently relax the tension and invite fluidity back into the tissues so that you can more easily palpate the organs.

4. Clear the large intestine (10 minutes)
5. Relax and open the area in the inguinal space (in front of the ASIS) and pubic bone. Encourage the tissues up toward the navel. Reposition the uterus if needed, and allow time for the ovaries and fallopian tubes to unwind. Relax any ligaments that are pulling on the right ovary and may be attached to the cecum (30 minutes)
6. Anchor the Lower Tan Tien (5 minutes)
7. Rest your hands on the belly, fill the organs with color (2 minutes)
8. Seal the client's Chi field and step away (2 minutes)

60 minutes

This treatment is beneficial for those with menstrual cramps, endometriosis, fibroids, pelvic pain, adhesions, back pain and infertility. If the ligament of Cleyet is pulled there can be pelvic irritation and even pain transmitted to the knees through the obturator foramen. Sink in slowly and deliberately to stretch this tissue. It may be bound up against the ovary.

During a woman's menstrual cycle, we do not work on those with endometriosis as it would irritate the tissues. Wait until menses has passed. Even young girls have pelvic pain. It is never too early to begin CNT treatments. Children will not need as long of a treatment, and are often not patient or relaxed enough for a 60-minute session. Keep them engaged with the use of color and sound. Make it a game for them.

Constipation

1. Clear, ground and charge your Chi Field (1 minute)
2. Direct the client's breath into their belly (5 minutes)

Observe where the restrictions are, if any, in their breath.
3. Soften the belly with a kneading, back and forth, movement (5 minutes)

If the connective tissue is very tight, take more time to gently relax the tension and invite fluidity back into the tissues so that you can more easily palpate the organs.

4. Clear the large intestine, repeat a few times (20 minutes)
5. Open the navel (10 minutes)
6. Open the eight windgates (10 minutes)
7. Anchor the Lower Tan Tien (5 minutes)
8. Rest your hands on the belly, fill the organs with color (2 minutes)
9. Seal the client's Chi field and step away (2 minutes)

60 minutes

Many people of all ages suffer with Constipation. Taking probiotics daily and eating a diet that includes fruits and vegetables will assist the large intestine to find its rhythm. The large intestine needs some bulk to move things along. However, using things like psyllium can irritate the lining of the gut, so use this sparingly. Moving and breathing are also important to our body's health and ability to metabolize food. Be sure to address any emotional holding in the body relating to the metal element.

Some people have multiple adhesions in their abdomen from injury, surgery and infections. Adhesions can limit the movement of any organ, and inhibit normal elimination. Work slowly and specifically to melt through adhesions, and teach your clients to do regular self CNT on their belly.

Irritable Bowel, SIBO, Crohns, Diverticulitis

1. Clear, ground and charge your Chi Field (1 minute)
2. Direct the client's breath into their belly (5 minutes)

Observe where the restrictions are, if any, in their breath.
3. Soften the belly with a kneading, back and forth, movement (5 minutes)

If the connective tissue is very tight, take more time to gently relax the tension and invite fluidity back into the tissues so that you can more easily palpate the organs. IF THERE IS PAIN WORK VERY GENTLY.

4. Clear the large intestine (10 minutes)
5. Rest your hands on the belly and feel the temperature and subtle movements of the small intestine. Starting near the navel, make small circles with your finger in an ever widening spiral pattern until you have covered the area of the small intestine (20 minutes)
6. Open the eight windgates gently with your fingers, not elbow (15 minutes)
7. Rest your hands on the belly, fill the organs with color (2 minutes)
8. Seal the client's Chi field and step away (2 minutes)

60 minutes

We are learning more about diet and pain every year. Individuals with irritable bowel, or SIBO, have a lower pain threshold than other clients and will need a light touch.

The application of Chi Nei Tsang treatments to client needs is unlimited. Each time I work with a client I find that the basic treatment techniques work very well for a wide variety of complaints. There may be more focus on a specific organ system, or emotional issue, however, the interaction of your hands and the client's intentional awareness is magical.

In class we discuss many specific needs, and it is not possible to list them all here. Every belly is unique to the individual. Your belly is not like anyone else's. Please contact me if you have questions about specific treatment issues.

Working with Color and Sound

Taoist Color Healing

In the previous treatment maps you see that I have included color as a final step in the healing session. Color is very toni-fying to the organs and restores them to their original vibration. We are using the wisdom of the five elements. Color and sound are ancient archetypes of healing and the body definitely responds to them. Be mindful of sounds and colors in your living space.

Each of us has a dominate sense; taste, touch, hearing, smell, sight. All of these senses live as high sense perception in the Chi Field. You may excel at seeing color, or feeling temperature coming from various parts of the body, or hearing vibration as guidance. I am able to feel the location and level of pain in a client's body. Not sure where this ability came from, but after a lifetime of putting my hands on clients, I became aware of this gift and confirmed it with many clients.

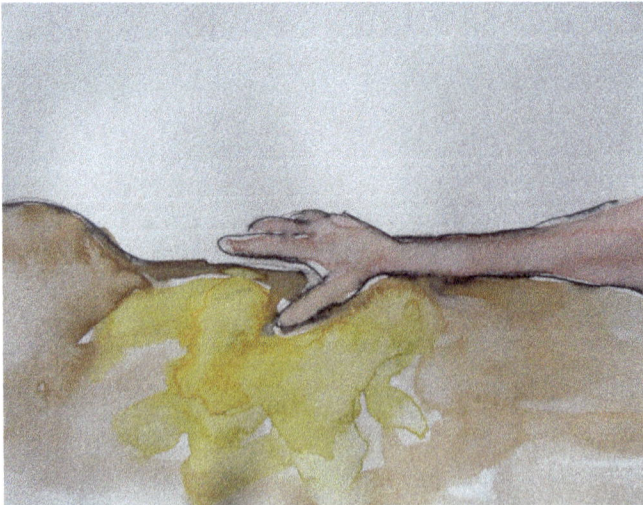

Earth element is a honey gold. Stomach, pancreas, esophagus, mouth, and here we will add the duodenum

Metal element is white, like the sun glinting off of polished metal. Lungs and large Intestine

Water element is dark blue. Kidneys and bladder

Wood element is spring green. Liver and gallbladder

Fire element is red. Heart and small intestine

Endocrine glands are a deep violet. Pineal gland, pituitary gland, thyroid, thymus, pancreas, adrenal, ovaries and testes.

Taking a few moments at the end of a session to visualize color filling the organ that you were helping is a peaceful transition away from hands on healing. You can also enlist the participation of the client in this practice, and it then becomes a teaching moment, or a suggestion of what the client may do for themselves at home. This is empowering and fun.

Taoist Sound Healing

The Six Healing Sounds meditation is a classic Taoist healing meditation. Anything that we can use to cultivate the quality and quantity of our own chi can be projected for a client's healing. You may have the high sense perception of sound healing and not only feel but see sound vibrations, like ripples across a still pond.

Sounds can be subvocal and barely audible, or loud and resonant. Loud sounds will break up stagnation, and softer sounds will ripple through the chi field like a gentle breeze. You must decide which is most appropriate for the person you are working with.

If a disease process has embedded itself deeply within the tissues of the body, then a loud sound is called for. If a distortion in the chi field has been created by an emotional response then a softer sound is effective.

Ancient Taoist practitioners treated the human body like an empty stalk or reed. The vibration of sounds and emotions creates an internal wind which we will study in depth in CNT 2. Review the six healing sounds with your instructor.

The Six Healing Sounds is unique because it includes the endocrine glands as one of the body systems which can be harmonized with sound. *HEEEEEE* is the high vibration sound which connects all of the endocrine glands. This is especially important for women of all ages.

In the following graph you can see the time periods when our bodies are most active within each organ system. There is a time of day for the Endocrine glands between 7pm and 11pm each evening.

The color to tonify the endocrine glands is a deep purple, like the color which emanates from the North Star.

TIMETABLE OF MERIDIANS

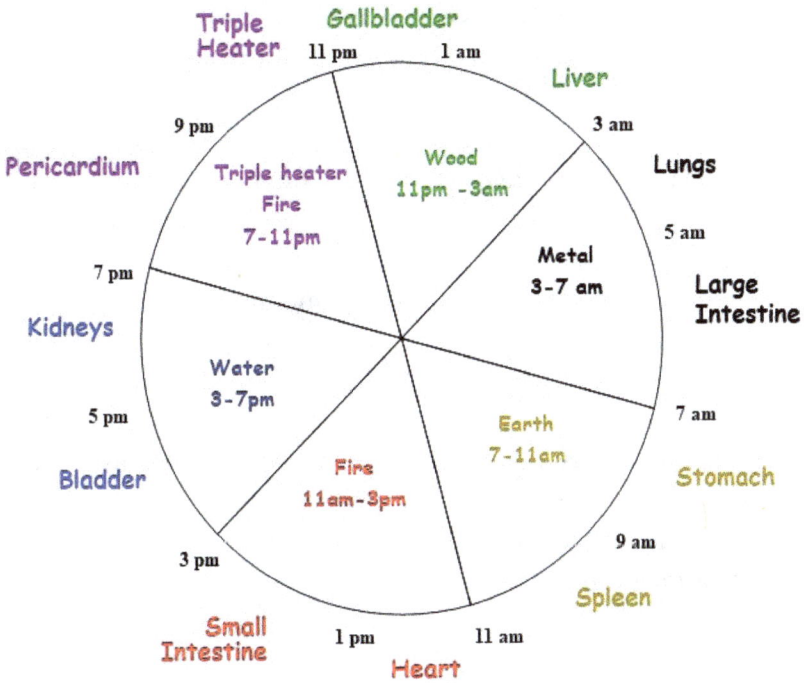

Thai Herbs

We use steamed Thai herbs made into a poultice during class, and during treatments. They are warming and fit very nicely into a Chi Nei Tsang treatment. I soak the herb bundles ahead of time and steam them for one hour in a vegetable steamer. The dried and chopped herbs are wrapped in muslin cloth and tied at the top. The classic herbal combination that I use from Thailand includes lemongrass, ginger, galangal, camphor, dried eucalyptus, peppermint, turmeric and kaffir lime. The combination of these herbs is very fragrant, which is wonderful for lung congestion, and produces a deeply penetrating and clearing action on the belly. Use caution with the steamed bundles, they are very hot and may need to be wrapped in a towel until they are safe to handle. The herbs can be used at any time during a treatment depending on what action you want. They can help to warm and relax the belly prior to massage with your hands, or they can be used at the middle and end of a CNT treatment to soothe and prolong the benefit of your treatment.

Self-Care for the Practitioner

The Six Healing Sounds

The practice of the six healing sounds for nourishing a healthy life has a long oral and written history. During the Qin Dynasty (221-207 BC) there was a record of this practice, and in the Han Dynasty (207 BC- 220 AD) we find written records buried in tombs. In the Tang dynasty (618-906AD) Sun Si Miao, and esteemed TCM doctor, wrote in the "Song of Hygiene" about the six healing sounds and outlined their specific benefits to the internal organs and their associated sense organs.

Healing practices that were passed down orally for centuries were eventually recorded on silk and bamboo and later unearthed in tombs. Many modern-day practitioners in China know of this practice and when I was in China in 2011 I met a Taoist Abbot who told me that this was, indeed, an advanced practice. He stressed the need to make the sounds gently and sub-vocally. Clearly the most basic practices are advanced practices, affording the practitioner immediate internal alchemical results. This is a classic Taoist foundation practice in that the simplest of practices become the most profound.

This practice is flexible and adaptable to each individual's needs. You may practice them in order, starting with wood and proceeding through the creation cycle, ending with the endocrine or triple burner sound, or only practice the sounds you need to treat specific conditions in the body. I like to focus my practice seasonally, meaning that in spring I would give specific focus to the wood element and the liver sound.

Many esteemed Taoist sages advised that the first step in practice is to subdue one's emotions, and then to harmonize the mind.

Chen Tuan marks these as the first three of 12 steps to attain the Tao.

Sun Buer
Be free from grief and anxiety.
A solitary cloud and wild crane beyond constraint.
Within a thatched hut,
Leisurely read the golden books.
Forests and streams outside the window,
At the edge of the rolling hills, water and bamboo.
Luminous moon and clear wind;
Become worthy to be their companion.

Taoist practitioners realize that humans have desires and emotions, however they provided us with alchemical formulas to transform this energy into pure chi.

As a healing practice the Six Healing Sounds meditation is unequaled in its ability to identify dense emotional energy/chi in the body; specifically in each organ, and to then diffuse it and break up patterns of stagnation which form disease and behavior problems. Communicating with color and sound to clear and tonify the organ's chi is a very old archetype of healing. You are connecting to the subtle energy/chi field by using your ability to visualize and guide the chi with sound and color. This practice recycles chi into its original pure form therefore bringing balance and harmony back into the body mind as it was in a primordial state.

If you are restoring your health it is important for every cell to be functioning at a high level of clarity, unencumbered with emotional toxins. The environment of the cell, the cell wall, is affected by your thoughts, emotions, and sounds. Women, pay close attention to the sounds and color used in this practice for balancing and strengthening the endocrine glands.

Sound and color are ancient archetypes of healing. Sound breaks up stagnation and patterns of disease, in this case stuck emotions. Color tonifies the cells of the body. True colors signify vibrant health. Reference the five elements graph on page 96 to see the colors (the metal element color is white). We begin the Six Healing Sounds meditation with the Inner Smile practice which lifts the frequency in the cells to a higher vibration. Then visual-ize each organ filling with a pure color that is associated with its element. The sounds will purge any low vibration emotions from the body – the sounds are always sub vocal, like a whisper. For the fire element the sound is *Haaaaa*. Feel the it emanating from the heart and small intestines, removing stagnation. The sound for the Earth element is *Hoooooo*, very guttural. The metal element sound is *Sssssssss*. The water element sound is *Chooooooooo*, like a wave crashing. Feel the contraction in your core around the kidneys as you make this sound. The wood element sound is *Shhhhhhhhh*. And the 6th healing sound is for the endocrine glands; pituitary, pineal, thyroid, thymus, adrenal, pancreas, ovaries and testes. The color which will tonify them is a deep night sky violet/purple. The sound is *Heeeeeeeee*. The virtuous behavior that comes from balanced en-docrine glands is effortless and harmonious communication.

Practice in class with a teacher, or listen to the CD which is included in this manual. You may want to watch it the first time through (track one on the CD). Both tracks are real time medita-tions. Practice at least once a day, more if you are recovering from illness. Doing the six healing sounds before bedtime is excellent for harmonizing the organs' chi and assisting you to sleep peace-fully. Do this meditation daily to clear your body/mind of low vibrations.

This is a foundation practice which will prepare you for other practices.

The graph on the next page explains which organs manifest specific emotions. It also shows you which color is used to tonify the organs (the color used to tonify the Metal element is White). The second graph will show you which seasons are associated with the organs.

The endocrine glands are included in the six healing sounds, and in the 24-hour meridian cycle they are active in the late evening, but have no season. The meridians and timetable of endocrine activity is shown in the final of the three graphs.

Taoists considered the hormones to be spirit molecules; very fine and very powerful, and were therefore given the color purple to match the North Star.

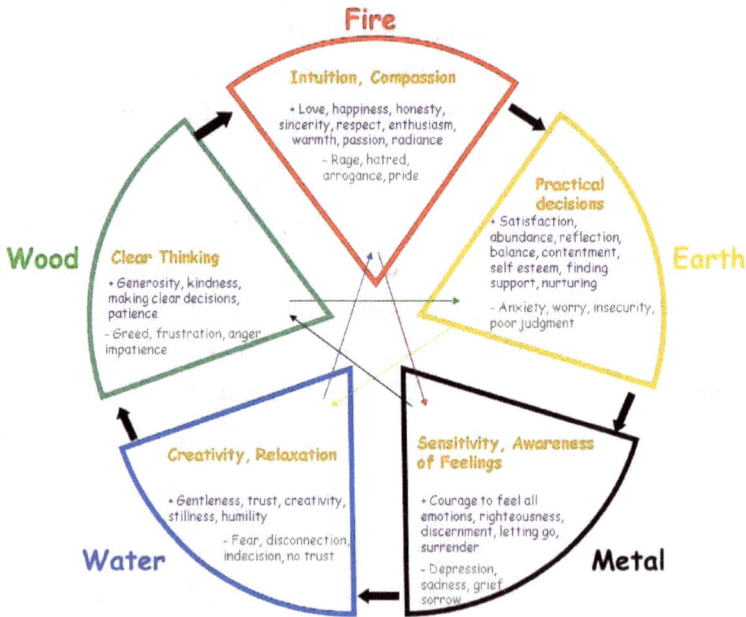

Positive emotions in purple, negative emotions in brown.
Orange signifies the mental state of being and behaviors that come from having balanced emotions.

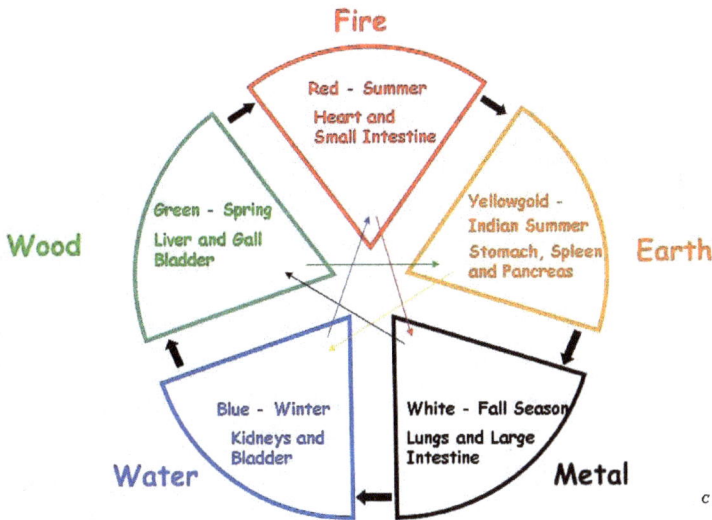

The five elements wheel showing:
- **Fire** — Red - Summer, Heart and Small Intestine
- **Earth** — Yellowgold - Indian Summer, Stomach, Spleen and Pancreas
- **Metal** — White - Fall Season, Lungs and Large Intestine
- **Water** — Blue - Winter, Kidneys and Bladder
- **Wood** — Green - Spring, Liver and Gall Bladder

C 2001 Caryn Diel

The five seasons and the five elements as they relate to the paired organs. It is wise to be mindful of the organs during their associated season. Nurture them with the proper foods and qigong practices. Slow down in the winter, rest more.

The Six Healing Sounds practice is useful in healing and it is also a Long Life/Yang Shen practice. One of my teachers, Master Mantak Chia, claims that this practice will cool down the organs' chi and allow the body to be more at ease. Emotions affect the organs, and unhealthy organs create unhealthy emotions.

Qigong

Many of our beautiful flowing Qigong forms have been handed down from masters and today we are discovering how to balance our lives with some very simple, yet powerful meditative movements.

Qigong is moving meditation. Let's take a look at the word Qigong. It is made up of two Chinese characters; Qi or Chi, meaning air, or a universal energy that permeates and flows thru everything; the breath that we all breathe, and Gong, which represents the effort or practice of learning to interact with chi and cultivate it for healing.

Qigong is a meditative practice of moving chi through and around the body to affect balance and better health.

"The ancient Chinese sages or Wu created Qigong as a life science system to maintain the health of the body, mind, and spirit. It stems from classical Daoist traditions and is rooted in the principles of Classical Chinese Medicine. In its true form, Qigong is a practice for cultivating knowledge and a main method for moving into Tian Ren He Yi (the state of oneness of the universe and the human being). Qigong is translated into English as 'Qi cultivation' or 'to work with the Qi.' There are many forms of Qigong practice: sitting meditation, movement (including Taijiquan and other internal martial arts), breath work, regulation of mental focus and emotions, visualizations, mudras, and mantras. The proper use of herbal supplements and food choices can be associated with Qigong. Cultivation of the classical arts – such as calligraphy and music – is considered a form of Qigong when conducted in a mindful manner. In any case, all the different forms have the same three keys, or three alignments: regulating the posture, regulating the breath, and regulating the mind. Qigong facilitates the development of a deeper relationship with Qi. This relationship helps the practitioner understand the laws of the universe and how they influence human life." (Master Zhongxian Wu)

There are probably thousands of Qigong forms, many developed specifically by individuals to heal certain ailments. There are martial forms of Qigong like Bone Breathing, or Bone Marrow Washing and Tan Tien Qigong which come from the Iron Shirt Tradition. There are spiritual forms of Qigong like Primordial Qigong and dream practices. The alchemical branch of Qigong includes meditations such as the Inner Smile and Six Healings Sounds, Microcosmic Orbit, and Fusion of the Five Elements. And there are Medical Qigong forms, like the ones I learned at the Xi Yuan hospital in Bejing which balance the organs energy. And there are specific forms to strengthen the liver, like Jade Woman.

Many Qigong forms include slow meditative movements, yet the most advanced forms do not require movement, only the directing of the chi through the organs and meridians of the body, to affect balance of chi flow for optimum health.

Chi takes on many qualities. It can be vibrant and of high quality or stagnant and charged with low level energy. We individually live with chi that is either enlivening and in balance, in excess or deficient. With conscious practice, observation and quiet reflection we can learn to evaluate and work with our chi level and how it flows through our bodies.

We gather chi from the air, food, water and from sleeping. Our thoughts and emotions also affect the quality of chi. Qigong practice teaches us to purify, cultivate, circulate, store and project chi for healing. As we become still like the practitioners of the past, we become more attuned to where we are out of flow, or out of balance.

As we move gently with Qigong, the breathing becomes deeper and the mind quiets. The blood shifts back into a more balanced pH. which allows for deeper meditation. Life events and emotions become less intense as the body and its glands and organs find new balance and fill with the higher virtues that we were born with.

With simple and consistent practice, we begin to cultivate life, and return our energy to pure source and the realm of primordial awareness.

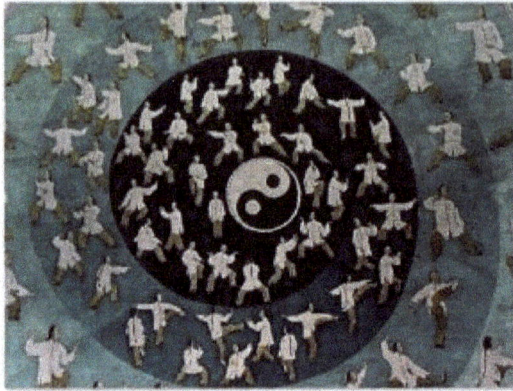

How do Seasonal Qigong Forms Support Your Health and Vitality?

Humans are nature. Our rhythms move naturally with the movement of the sun, moon, (light and dark) planets and stars, tides and rivers, the flowering and fruiting of plants, the movement of animals and birds. Even the digestion of our foods is dependent on what is available each season. Everything that we need to know about our world and keeping healthy can be found simply or metaphorically in nature.

Our breath is just right for a human body. The respiration of a tree is just right for the tree. Both have consciousness and ways of communicating. The planet has one breath each year, an inhale and an exhale. Drawing in chi and letting go of chi as the earth moves on its axis. The hummingbird has a quick movement, the galaxies a much slower movement.

Qigong movements create a flow of chi through the body and its structure, the meridians. Each meridian is a river of chi moving between the interior and the exterior of the body, from organs to the extremities and back. Every organ has its season, sound, and color, and time of day. And therefore, we can use qigong to strengthen the organs and our overall health by choosing a movement which recognizes the organ and brings more chi into the organ. Sound and color produce a quality of chi. Movement creates a flow of chi.

For example, during the spring it is a great idea to choose movements that clear and tonify the liver chi. Locate the liver and gallbladder meridians and make some movements, or do some stretches and massage for the liver and gallbladder meridians. Make it fun. And send some vibrant spring green color from your mind's eye into the liver and gallbladder to tonify them. Sounds will break up stagnation and move out stuck chi. Try the sound *Shhhh* and see the old chi moving out of your liver to be recycled by the universe.

Now you have a spontaneous Qigong form.

Each season/element has a movement. Winter/Water brings us to a still point; a place of rest and rejuvenation. When we give ourselves the gift of stillness our entire being has an opportunity to become refreshed. Winter Qigong forms that I teach focus on slow movements to open the kidney and bladder meridians, and have longer quiet sitting meditations. I allow the natural darkness to fill the room. Pearl of the Night is a Winter Qigong form that I created. It is very simple and restorative.

Spring/Wood begins the movement upward and outward like the sap rising in the trees, stimulated by the wind moving the woods. Traditionally we use this time of year to detoxify our bodies. Nature, and our liver, is pushing chi up and out through branches and meridians. Qigong forms that stimulate the liver are great for spring. I like forms like Swimming Dragon which open the spine and Jade Woman which clears liver chi.

Bone Breathing Qigong

For thousands of years the Chinese have used various forms of Qigong exercise to realize better health. Bone Breathing is also referred to as Iron Shirt Qigong, due to its association with the warrior monks (martial artists) in China and their use of this form to create a dense reservoir of chi in their bones, which established a strong layer of wei chi at the level of the skin.

Bone Breathing Qigong, a Taoist practice, is a practical way to increase the strength of the bones and the vitality of the blood. This active meditation is representative of the finest in Taoist alchemy. With continued practice one may realize many benefits and positively shift blood enzymes to healthy levels; boosting immunity by bringing universal chi into the blood cells. Bones are relatively porous, and are therefore always "breathing". Bones are believed to vibrate like hollow reeds.

The effects of Bone Breathing Qigong are many. The practice prevents bone loss, reverses osteoporosis, speeds healing, boosts the immune system, positively affects blood enzymes and increases your reserve of chi. After the chi gathers in the deepest part of the bone marrow it can expand out to the level of the skin. This creates a protective layer of chi, called wei chi, which protects the body from invasion of negative chi and germs. Wei chi is what protects you when there is a change of weather, and the climate penetrates into the body creating damaging winds. Some references refer to this qigong form as Bone Marrow Washing. Indeed, the visualization and directing of chi through the bone marrow resembles a washing action. I like to imagine the ocean surf moving in and out of the bones.

"The practice of bone breathing was introduced into the Western world by the Taoist teacher Mantak Chia back in 1983. One of the first students was a middle aged woman residing in Los Angeles, California who was losing bone mass in her spine at an alarming rate. She was under the care of several specialists who had been unable to arrest the bone loss. The predicted outcome of her illness would be a spinal collapse threatening the nervous system and bringing paralysis or early death. As soon as she heard about bone breathing she enrolled in a class and began a daily routine of 3 hours of continuous exercise bringing subtle breath to the bone marrow. Since the skeleton is considered an antenna, the most efficient way of practicing bone breathing is standing up in a special posture that allows the complete skeleton to be aligned in the most efficient way with the flow of universal energies.

Within six months of practice she not only arrested bone mass loss but also began reversing the process and gained some 10% of the mass back. The doctors who had been treating her were at a loss to explain the reversal. Within three years of continued practice she began to appreciably regain bone mass and at the end of five years had replaced 100% her bone mass without indications that there had ever been osteoporosis.

This case is not an isolated one. Since the 1980's, similar cases have been reported by practitioners in different countries in Europe and the Americas. Bone breathing has been successfully used also for accelerated healing of broken bones and torn ligaments. An important condition in bone breathing practice is being able to feel the area being worked with the attention. The ancient Taoists have left us the maxim that says that 'The practice of the Tao begins with feeling'. Without feeling the practice may degenerate into being just a mental exercise unrelated to the bones." (Juan Li)

This type of Qigong would be considered Medical Qigong for its ability to bring chi into the red and white blood cells in the bones. Red blood cells are formed in the long bones of the femur, humerus, and tibia. White bloods cells form in the flat bones of the pelvis sternum and skull. When we are born our bones are heavy with circulation. As we age the bones become fatty and brittle. Bone Breathing Qigong practice can prevent and reverse this thinning of the bones. It is a fine example of a Yang Shen, longevity practice, as well as a healing and curing practice.

Like many of our historical references, the personal stories of the success of Bone Breathing Qigong are anecdotal and not peer-reviewed scientific studies. However, the desired result will happen if one practices regularly with clear intention. I personally have felt a huge boost in my energy levels throughout the day when I have done Bone Breathing. And I have seen students with broken bones heal quickly using this practice when all other methods failed. A student of mine who practices acupuncture in New York found that her cancer patients experienced relief from neuropathy when they listened to the Bone Breathing Qigong CD. This is a great example of a practice which enhances our immune system and shifts blood enzymes. Another student of mine shared this with her friend while he was in the hospital. After one session the hospital staff discovered inadvertently that his liver enzymes had changed for the better. And there are more success stories from around the world.

In Traditional Chinese Medicine the term marrow (Sui) is considered the substance that is the common matrix of bones, bone marrow, spinal cord and brain. Marrow circulates chi and irrigates the bones. The Chinese character for Sui is composed of the combination of images below. Bone on the upper left, flesh and tissues on the lower left, lower right image depicts the idea of building something and something walking aside the building. This represents the movement of marrow inside the bones. Marrow nourishes the bones, spinal cord and the brain.

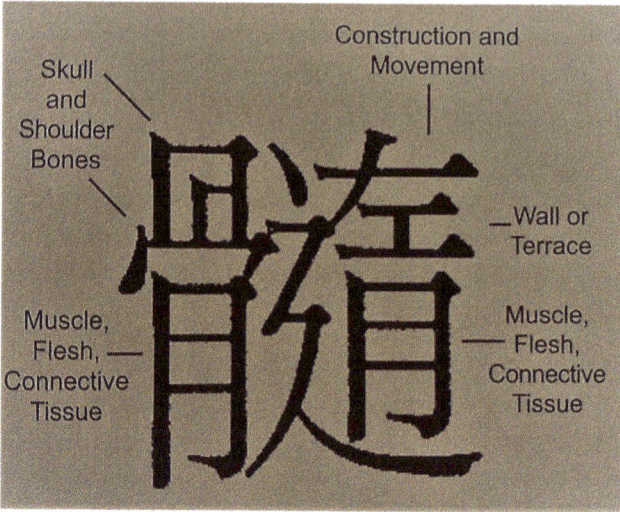

Image from J. A. Johnson, Chinese Medical Qigong Therapy

This practice can be done standing, sitting or lying down. If you practice standing you become solidly grounded and strengthen your ability to direct chi through your skeletal system. The more grounded you are the more the chi rises up. If you are not feeling well, sitting is the best posture.

It is invigorating and a good practice to do on a daily basis, a practical and profound method of Medical Qigong. For both women and men Bone Breathing Qigong is especially good for maintaining healthy marrow. Therefore, it is included in both the curing and healing practices as well as the prevention and longevity practices.

Breath, Visualization and Posture.

Using your breath and your ability to visualize is where this begins. If you are standing find a comfortable stance with soft knees. I like to begin by moving with my breath, sinking on the inhale and standing up and pushing my palms toward the earth on the exhale. This gentle up and down movement keeps me relaxed as I breathe and guides the chi into the bones. If you are sit-ting our laying down, begin by connecting with your breath in a focused way on the inhale and exhale. This does not have to be a really big breath, just a conscious breath.

Open your chi field to the primordial chi field of infinite source. Connect with the highest, purest source of chi that you can imagine, and beyond.

We enlist our ability to visualize, which may seem like simple a mental practice, yet it is one of our strongest allies in self-healing. Many Taoist practices seem to begin with a mental approach, but actually this gives the mind a job, allows you to focus, and even-tually the mind gets out of the way. To affect healing, Chi needs guiding and purifying. What happens is that we gradually begin to feel the chi moving in the bones. Some chi sensations are pleas-ant, and some are not. If the chi has been blocked in an area on your bones, you may feel nothing, or you may feel warmth and tingling, or a jolting sensation. Every one of us is different every time we practice. I was practicing Bone Breathing the day after I injured my leg and knee playing tennis. The chi shot through my leg like a lightning rod and straightened it out.

Now that you are connected to pure Universal Chi, bring your attention to the tips of your toes, all ten toes, and imagine that there are openings like straws at the tips of all your toes. Invite pure chi to enter the small bones of your toes on the inhale, swirling, stimulating and clearing out the marrow. On the exhale release the old chi. Continue bringing in fresh chi and releasing old chi on each breath. Do this for several breaths before moving on. If you are doing this alone you may want to look at a picture of the skeleton before you begin to refresh your memory of the many bones in your body. There are approximately 200 bones.

You can imagine the chi as a color if this helps you to visualize. I picture the chi moving in and out like the waves coming in on a shoreline and retreating with the old chi. I enjoy this image as an example of bone marrow washing.

Continue breathing and visualizing the chi moving up the toes to the feet, ankles, legs, knees, femur, hips, pelvis, spine, and ribs. Take your time in each location and notice what you feel, or if there is a lack of feeling.

Now bring your attention to your fingertips. All ten fingers. Breathe into the small bones of the fingers trying to imagine the shape of the bones and the bone marrow. Continue to the bones of the hands, wrists, forearms, elbows, humerus, shoulder, scapula, clavicle, head, jaw and teeth.

Now you are breathing into all of the bones of the body at once. Continue with a few more breaths and then rest. Notice how your body is moving through space. Notice if you feel more grounded and present. Are your bones feeling heavy?

After several months of this practice you can begin Bone Packing. I will cover this in another chapter that will lead you into the practice of Buddha Palms.

When one feels the resiliency of strong, supple bones and a cheerful vitality exuding from the blood, self-esteem improves and the quality of life experiences are enhanced to their fullest enjoyment.

*The Bone Breathing CD that I have recorded is beneficial in many ways. It is great for improving one's overall vitality, and is also very effective *for those healing from diseases and chemotherapy because it can be done lying down. It improves the regeneration of bone marrow and bone strength, and strengthens the immune system.*

Tao Yin

Tao Yin (or Dao in) is the Chinese word for physical energy directing. Using one's mind-eye-heart we direct chi for opening the flow through the Meridians, thereby bringing ease of movement to the body, and a balanced interaction between the organs of the physical body.

Thousands of years ago the people living by the Yellow River developed movement practices to enhance a healthy and long life. People lived simply, they sat but had no chairs, they ate but had no tables. Just as we experience today, too much repetition can create stagnation, poor health and pain. For thousands of years people have been guiding chi.

> "Transformation of human society comes from intuitive genius which sees design, beauty and harmony for the individual in relation to people, to earth, and to heaven, which can be expressed and taught.
>
> Teachings recording such genius were attributed to Huang Di, The Yellow Emperor and his ministers. Chinese legend says Huang Di reigned from 2696 to 2598 B.C. He was third in the line of great men who helped to create the civilizations of China." (Ling Shu, 1993 translated by Wu Jing-Nuan, page xi)

Huang Di asks one of his ministers, Qi Bo, about the meridians of the human body. His response is that there are six celestial vibration patterns and from these arise the Yin and Yang meridian system. The twelve meridians correlate with the twelve months of the year and the twelve (two hour) time periods of the day. The organs in the human body resonate with the Dao when chi in the meridians flows freely.

Wise people like Chen Tuan developed postures to counter repetition and bring more fluidity into the mind and body. He was also mindful of the movement of the seasons and developed movements that harmonized the human body with the body of nature. Some of these movements appear to mimic the movements of animals, others look like yoga postures. The five animals we see imitated in Tao Yin are the tiger, deer, bear, monkey and the bird. All Tao Yin postures are meant to gently stretch open the meridians while not overstressing any joints or ligaments, as compared to Indian Yoga which focuses on opening the Chakras. Using your breath to complete the extension of chi is key to making these movements successful and enjoyable. Hold a pose for 5 or more breaths, being certain not to create any pain. Allow the breath to move into the meridian and guide the chi to move with your mind's eye.

In modern day terms we could say that this type of gentle exercise will reduce stress and energy blockages. Tao Yin is an excellent practice to do at the end of a day to bring balance to repetitive postures that you have held. It is also a great warmup in the morn-ing to enliven the body before you start your day. Tao Yin can be done by anyone, at any age, and with all health backgrounds. It is very gentle and can be done sitting or lying on the floor, or sitting in a chair. In China, Tao Yin is prescribed for healing and preven-tion of disease. Among Daoist practitioners self massage and Tao Yin are a common practice after long periods of sitting medita-tion. Enjoy the benefits of Tao Yin if you have been sitting too long at a desk, standing for work, have been ill and lying down a lot, riding in a car, or sitting a long time in meditation.

A record of many Tao Yin moves is found in the Taoist Canon which was compiled in China between 1436 and 1449 A.D. Dur-ing the Tang Dynasty 652 ad, Tao Yin became an official part of

Court Medicine. The famous physician, Sun Simiao (581-682 AD) compiled "Prescriptions of a thousand ounces of gold" in which he outlined many qigong and tao yin prescriptions.

Chen Tuan (born 870 A.D.) was a student of Li He, who was a student of Yin Xi, and Yin Xi was a direct student of LaoTzu. Chen Tuan is known as the dreaming priest, he perfected Taoist Dream practice and sometimes slept for hundreds of days at a time. He was also a respected sage who performed divination practices at the court for emperors. His chi had to be clear and supple to achieve all that he did. The gentle stretching postures of Tao Yin allow fluidity to return to the connective tissue which encompasses the meridians.

Lao Tze (500 bc) called it regulating the respiration. Some say the Lao Tzu lived to be 260 years old. Lao Tzu says in chapter 76 of the Tao te Ching,

When people are alive,
Their bodies are soft and supple.
When people die,
They are stiff and hardened.
When tree, grass and animals are alive,
They are soft and pliable.
When they are dead
They become dry and brittle.

Tao Yin:

1. Harmonizes and guides the chi through the mind/body
2. Supports the tendons and joints
3. Relaxes the psoas and diaphragm
4. Improves flexibility
5. Releases toxins via the breath
6. Strengthens the lower tan tien

You do not need to know all of the meridians to receive the benefits of Tao Yin. Guide the chi with your intention, and it will move during the resting phases. Chi, or energy, is able to be guided like this. Your active intention and each posture initiates the yang phase and uses the breath to stretch the body. The resting yin phase allows the chi to move where you have guided it. Take a resting breath or two between postures and enjoy the feeling of chi flowing in your body. Your spirit will be more content when your body is relaxed. Breathe deeply by letting the abdomen expand on the inhale and pull up the perineum on the exhale, in this way you strengthen the lower tan tien.

Hua Ching Ni says to imagine you have been lying in a cave for a thousand years, you are completely relaxed and as you wake up you realize that you are a spirit who has awakened in a physical body. You take a deep breath and begin to make physical movements. There is no rush, slowly turn your attention to the life force in your body.

There are many postures and movements that you can choose from, it is not necessary to do them all. The goal is to rebalance your chi and harmonize your mind and body. Imitate the flow of water, or bamboo moving in the wind. Sit like a tiger resting in the grass, and stretch like a dragon reaching for heaven. I have written the following for you as an easy introduction to some of the Tao Yin postures.

Begin with Conscious Breathing. Lying on your back, smile and breathe in golden light to your face, heart and lower tan tien. Place your hands gently on your belly and feel the expansion of your breath. Then place your hands on your chest and feel the movement of breath here. As you move into each posture, stay there for three to five breaths.

1. Pericardium and Kidney meridians

Laying on your back. Flex the soles of your feet and make a fist as you inhale. Press your fingers into the Lao Gong point in the middle of your palm as you make the fist. Guide the chi up from the bottom of your feet to flow around the heart. As you exhale relax your fists and relax the feet. The chi flows back down and out the soles of the feet. Sometimes this is called the Lotus Fire and Water meditation. Imagine the sun above your head filling your heart, and the water below you coming into the soles of your feet to fill the kidneys. Your heart is the lotus flower and your kidneys are the lotus bulbs.

2. Kidney and Bladder Meridians

Stretch out like a starfish with your hands above your head and your legs open like a V. Stretch one arm, then one leg, the other arm, then the other leg so that you open the space around the kidneys. As you reach out in all four directions you open the space around your kidneys for chi to flow in. This is a wonderful stretch for anyone who is yin deficient or having hot flashes.

Bring knees up toward your chest and reach thru the knees to grab the ankles. Let the legs fall open to stretch the kidney meridian.

Hug your knees into your chest and gently rock from side to side.

Sit up with legs straight, and spine lifted up. Move your chin toward your toes to stretch the bladder meridian.

3. Liver and Gallbladder

Sit with both legs extended to the front, opened into a V as widely as is comfortable. Do not raise the knees, but keep them attached to the floor. Keeping the spine erect (not rounded) reach forward until you feel a stretch in the liver meridian.

Lying on your back again, bring the knees up to the chest, hug them in and then let them fall to one side, stretching the GB meridian. Arms rest flat on the floor and the head looks away from the bent legs. Then let them fall to the other side as the head looks the opposite direction.

4. Lung and Large Intestine.

Standing or kneeling or sitting, clasp hands together behind the back and lean back, looking up. Then come forward bending to the floor with the arms and shoulders opening forward, hands are still clasped. Change thumb position and try it again. Three deep breaths

Cross your legs in a seated position and reach both hands over your head. Turn your palms to face the sky. Look up.

5. Spleen, Stomach and Pancreas.

Fold one leg in front of you and stretch one leg out behind you like a tail. Keep the spine moving forward (pigeon pose). Change to the other leg. Take three deep breaths.

Lying face down on your belly, place your hands flat on the floor near your shoulders. Push yourself up so that your chest is lifted but your hips still face and touch the floor. Look up.

6. Heart and Small Intestine.

Sit with legs open wide, the knees bent and the soles of the feet together. Hold the hands around the toes, and bring the feet in toward the body as much as possible. Then, slowly bend forward trying to touch the forehead toward the thumbs.

With the same leg position, lean forward and look to one side, twisting the spine. Then look to the other side.

7. Hip Opener. *Preparation for sitting meditation*

Cross your legs and arms and bend your head toward the floor. Breathe, and change the leg and arms positions, to fold over again. As you come up into a seated position you will feel your sits bones balanced on the floor.

Gently shift your awareness inside to your breath for meditation.

Chi Nei Tsang Self Massage

1. Lie down on your back in a comfortable, quiet place. Bend your knees so that your back is relaxed and your feet are flat on the floor. Put a few pillows under your knees to support them in this relaxed position.

2. Place your hands on your belly and breathe deeply, filing your abdomen first and then let the breath rise up into your lungs. Exhale completely and wait until the next breath comes naturally. Notice any places that hesitate to take in breath and chi. Observe any emotion that arises with the breath. Continue breathing with conscious awareness for several minutes.

3. Using your fingers, feel the texture of the skin inside the rim of your navel. Massage firmly in all directions inside the navel to about half of the depth of your navel. Allow time for the navel to shift and connect to all parts of your body via the connective tissue. Feel the energetic connections from your navel to other places in your body. You may use various methods of massage (circles, pulsing, or simply holding a stretch). Take as much time as you need, this may become a large segment of the self-massage.

4. Move your hands to the lower left quadrant of the abdomen and find the sigmoid and descending colon. Gently pump the large intestine with your fingers. This creates circulation,

hydration, intestinal transit and affects the movement of lymph of the pelvis.

5. Continue this technique along the entire length of the descending colon, transverse colon and ascending colon, ending at the cecum in the lower right quadrant of the abdomen. At the flexures of the intestine, under the rib cage on right and left sides, stretch the tissues down to create more space for the breath to move the diaphragm. If there is pain anywhere, pause and breathe, allowing the tissues to respond.

6. Explore areas of your belly that call out to you for attention and relaxation; if you have consistent complaints from your stomach, small intestine, liver and gallbladder, or anywhere else, then spend some time with your hands to massage gently and send healing chi into the area. You can rest your hands over these areas and do the Six Healing Sounds, or send color into the organs for healing.

7. Rest and return to your breath. Notice the changes that have occurred in your belly and your awareness. Smile.

Bibliography

Chia, Mantak. *Chi Nei Tsang*. Destiny Books. Rochester, Vermont. 1993

Johnson, Jerry Alan. *Chinese Medical Qigong Therapy*. The International Institute of Medical Qigong. Pacific Grove, California. 2002

Marin, Gilles. *Healing from Within with Chi Nei Tsang*. North Atlantic Books. Berkeley, California. 1999

Matsumoto, Kiiko and Stephen Birch. *Hara Diagnosis: Reflections on the Sea*. Paradigm Publications. Brookline, Massachusetts. 1988

Mochizuki, James Shogo. *Anma, The art of Japanese Massage*. Kotobuki Publications. Saint Paul, MN. 1995

Wu Jing-Nuan. *Ling Shu or The Spiritual Pivot*. University of Hawai'i Press. Honolulu, Hawaii. 1993

Author Caryn Boyd Diel

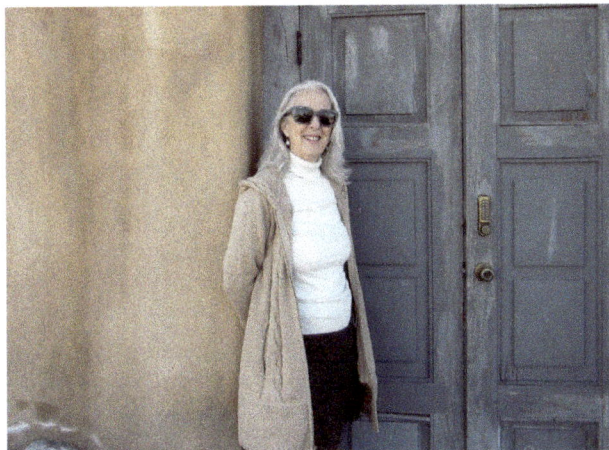

Caryn Boyd Diel is the founder and director of the White Cloud Institute. A graduate of the Barbara Brennan School of Healing and a Senior Healing Tao instructor, Caryn is able to move fluidly between the physical, emotional, mental, and spiritual bodies to assist clients and students to find new direction and wellness. She brings a compassionate understanding to the journey of healing and self-discovery.

Caryn enjoys teaching others how the human energy field contributes to health and the evolution of consciousness. Caryn combines cutting edge quantum physics with ancient Taoist teachings into her ever evolving curriculum. For more information on certification courses or continuing education visit the website: WhiteCloudInstitute.info

Caryn has been teaching Chi Nei Tsang classes around the world for 20 years. She has recorded several Qigong and Meditation CDs and DVDs and a three hour instructional DVD on Chi Nei Tsang fundamentals.

www.ingramcontent.com/pod-product-compliance
Lightning Source LLC
Chambersburg PA
CBHW061022220326
41597CB00017BB/2368